Tales from the Scales

MaryFran Clingan

Divine Intervention:

Mess on the Floor

Toaster Coffin

The Fat Dog

Love and Food

Drinks:

Stink Bug

The Death

The Switcheroo

Exercise:

Fool me once....

Self-Sacrificing Sister

Can You

Game On

The Wind Tunnel

Girls with Gears

Hiking with Snakes

You Get What You Pay for

You Actually Used It

Freight Train

Who Knew

Disc Breaks

First Ride

Trail of Tears

Trail of Tears Redux

Trail of Tears Onward

Tenderloin

The Double Stumble

An Easy Ride

Food:

Hoss's Cake

Pizza

Empress Chicken

A Rush

Chewing Gum

Save More Eat More

The Steakhouse Runs

Where's the Bread

Counting Chips

It's Not What you Eat

The Fickle Friend

But it's Zero

Sauerkraut Bomb

Divine Intervention

Divine intervention is a real thing that I have experienced in my weight loss journey. There comes a time (multiple times actually) when my motivation has been strong but my will power was weak. I want the end result so bad, yet find myself eating food that was not planned or skipping my planned exercise. Sometimes though, I have had the awesome experience of having a divine intervention that kept me from eating the food that would have sent me off course! I have had off the wall and random experiences that have given me the boost or motivation that I needed at that exact moment. I have had these divine interventions work in my favor to keep me on track, even when my will power had failed.

Mess on the Floor

I was doing really good with my weight loss efforts. I was on track with my eating for the day. I was watching everything I ate carefully. I knew exactly what I was eating the rest of the day in order to stay within my food budget. It was already tracked. I was set! Or was I set? Ok, I was only set only until my husband (ex) came home and said that he wanted to have pizza for dinner. What???? What was I going to do? I hadn't planned to eat pizza and pizza was not in my food budget in terms of calories. Was there really any question though? I made that pizza. I watched and calculated every ingredient. I practically counted every shred of cheese that went onto that pizza. I was careful with the whole process and calculated what it would cost my caloric budget. I knew that eating two pieces would cause me to go a bit overboard in terms of my food budget. Yet I had figured that I could squeak it into my daily food budget. Two pieces could work. No more! It wasn't the most optimal dinner but I figured that two pieces wouldn't mess me up too badly. I didn't think about my addictive, food loving side.   My word, when that pizza came out of the oven it smelled like heaven! Holy cow. I was actually salivating! I still held onto some vague idea that I could hold to my plan of eating 2 pieces of pizza.   I cut the pizza into slices and the cheese just oozed. Oh, the melted cheese! It melted my heart and my resolve. I couldn't resist. I slide some pizza onto my plate. One piece, two pieces, three pieces and four pieces of pizza went onto my plate! Four pieces? Where did my plan go? I justified it by telling myself that I would have gone back for the other two pieces anyway Because seriously, who wants to walk back to the kitchen to get more pizza? Not I! Obviously that thinking was the overweight MaryFran's thought process. I had already accepted the fact that my willpower had left me. The deed was completed. I was eating my half of that pizza. I picked up my plate and started to walk out of the kitchen. I don't know exactly what I did. But somehow, I bumped the plate of pizza. The plate wobbled and I watched in horror as two pieces of pizza slide off the plate and landed on the carpet.... upside down! My first moments of horror were as a result of seeing that cheesy saucy pizza laying on my carpet. Secondly, I thought about the loss of one half of my dinner. Very quickly though, I realized that this was a stroke of divine intervention. This was actually a good thing. Sure, I had to clean the carpet but there was NO temptation to eat those extra two pieces of pizza. I may have had a temporary lapse in wise weight loss decisions, but a simple accident put me right back on track!

Toaster Coffin

I love bread! I could eat bread in so many formats! Bread, rolls, biscuits, with butter, with jelly, toasted or untoasted. I love it all! I have a very difficult time controlling my portion sizes when it comes to toast. I could literally eat piece after piece of toast. It was with some trepidation that I popped my two pieces of bread into the toaster. I was so hungry for toast. I planned to keep my intake at two pieces. I knew that it was going to be a battle to keep from gorging on more and more pieces of toast! My mouth was salivating as the bread disappeared into the toaster.   Almost immediately I knew something was wrong. What was wrong? Well, it doesn't take a rocket scientist to realize that the rustling noise inside my toaster was abnormal! My eyes were wide when I heard a squeak Even worse, the squeak was coming from inside the toaster!   Then there was silence. The ensuing silence in the kitchen was deafening. With a mounting horror I realized what had happened. Unbeknownst to me, a mouse had gotten into my toaster and was having a breakfast of bread crumbs while I was preparing my breakfast. I stood there in horror.   Was the mouse going to run in freakish misery from my toaster? I didn't know what was going to happen so I did the only thing I could think of. I grabbed the toaster, ran to the door and whipped that toaster outside. I stood in the safety of my kitchen and watched that toaster. There was no movement. I got brave and moved outside (I really don't like mice!) I poked the toaster with my foot. There was no movement except for the partially toasted bread sliding out of the toaster.   Feeling bold, I peeked into the slots. Oh yes, there it was! A dead electrocuted mouse lay in the toaster coffin.   There was no toast eaten that day. The toaster coffin was thrown away! Traumatized, it was months before I even contemplated buying a new toaster. Even after I bought a new replacement toaster, I just seemed to have no appetite for toast. Eventually the love for toast was rekindled, but for a few months, divine intervention (if we can call the death of a mouse divine intervention) helped me to avoid the delicious pitfall in my weight loss journey. As a side note, I am still wary of toasters even after many years.

The Fat Dog

Over the years I had attempted to run. My standard thought was that, "you don't see fat runners". So, I kept trying to make myself a runner. It wasn't until about the 4th or 5th attempt to become a runner that I actually stuck with it and made it work. I was determined and I was focused. I started out running with a friend and we were both completing the couch to 5K program. We would do the bulk of our runs on our own, in our own time frame. But once a week we would meet up and run together. It was a great motivator. I did my scheduled runs so that I would be able to keep up with her as she also progressed through the couch to 5K program. It was a great set up and it worked well for both of us. It was very motivational and the accountability was fabulous!

There were some amazing benefits of running in the morning. I got to see the sunrise during my runs. I was able to breathe in the sounds and smells of nature while I was out. I also got to recognize the people that also utilized the same National Park (The Antietam Battlefield) that I used for my daily runs. In particular, I noticed an older man walking with his white overweight poodle. Every time I was out, I would see him. We nodded at each other but stayed focused on our own workouts.

However, it was on one of my solo runs that I had the most interesting encounter with him. I had reached the point in my training where I was to run for an extended period of time. I was honestly quite scared of that long stretch. For the plan I was following, that was a 20 minute stretch of time. I had never before run for 20 minutes at one time! NEVER! I was sure I would tank and not be able to complete it. I definitely had a mental block for this 20-minute run. But I was determined! I knew the couch to 5 k plan was solid so I kept telling myself to trust the plan. It also helped that I knew that my friend was also doing it and I didn't want to get left in the dust! When it was time to run, I started to run. It wasn't fast. It wasn't furious. It probably wasn't even pretty. But I was running. The minutes started to tick by. I was doing it! I kept running. I looked at my watch and I was at 18 minutes. At that point, I knew I had it in the bag! I was doing it! I started to cry. I was sobbing from not only my relief but also elation that I was actually doing it. I wasn't giving up though I still had two minutes to complete. I sobbed every step of those last two minutes!   When my timer went off to indicate that my run was done, I slowed to my fast-paced walk for my cool down (as per the program). I looked up and there stood the gentleman and his poodle. They were waiting for me along the side of the road where I would be walking in just a few moments. I smiled and shakily wiped my eyes. Afterall, I didn't want him to see me crying. I had pulled myself together by the time I walked up to where he was standing. His words sent me spiraling right back into a pit of emotional elation.

"I just wanted to tell you that I've watched you progress these last weeks and you are doing great!"

 Such a simple sentence. But his words meant so much to me! I stopped that day and chatted with him and petted his dog. It was one of the most uplifting experiences I have ever had with a stranger!

I kept running after that day. I actually ran consistently on the battlefield for the next few years. I never saw that man or dog again. They were truly my angels that day when I was so overcome with emotion at my accomplishment!   They were just what I needed that day.

Love and Food

I went to a wedding! Weddings are awesome. Love is in the air, as is the wonderful aroma of food! Yes, weddings are full of delicious food! The wedding I went to was gorgeous. The bride was beautiful and the food was excellent! I have been thrown off my weight loss course at weddings. They can be a pitfall for healthy eating. But this wedding? I was lucky that day.   The bride's father had apparently had a health scare and had changed his diet drastically. Because of that, they had some seemingly healthier options there! They had an appetizer table, which contained the normal appetizers but also a lot of fruit! I was able to fill up my plate with healthy options. Maybe a bit higher in calories than I was used to, but at least I was eating foods that were lower in calories and had nutritional value! I was also pleased that they had two options of cake. One of which was angel food. It made an easier choice for me. I was able to indulge in a piece of angel food cake instead of the higher calorie choice of red velvet cake with the wonderful icing! Which yes, the old me (or maybe the current internal me) would have loved the red velvet cake! I was so proud of myself for the choices that made that wedding!

Even with my good choices, I was worried when I got home the night of the wedding. I did something that I should never have done. I did step on the scale before I went to bed. Yes, I know, weigh yourself at the same time during the day. I usually do it in the morning! But even though I had chosen wisely, I still indulged in more calories/points than normal and I wanted to know if I had done any damage. I should have NEVER stepped on the scales. But I did and it looked as if I was back where I was about a week or so earlier. My decision to hop on the scale that evening gave myself a full night of worry and angst. Luckily, in the morning it was pretty much back in line in terms of my weight. I knew that I couldn't have two days of indulgences though, so I upped my exercise and watched my food intake carefully and I was able to have a significant loss at my weekly weigh in! The fact that they had healthy options at this wedding, divine intervention!

Drinks

One of my ongoing missions on my weight loss journey has been to drink my water. Water is beneficial to pretty much every bodily function and it aids in weight loss efforts by acting as a natural appetite suppressant. Admittedly, at times I have struggled with drinking enough water. But at other times, I have been a water drinking machine.   Of course there were mishaps and mayhem with my water consumption efforts!

Stink bug

I was sitting by my computer playing games, editing pictures and talking to friends. It was a nice quiet evening at home.   I had my trusty 64-ounce water jug/bottle sitting there beside me as I was working on reaching my daily goal of water consumption. I was in a good routine and habit with my water so I wasn't even thinking about drinking water as I absently reached for it and brought it to my lips. I tilted it back and opened up my mouth. Immediately I began to feel and hear a crackling in my mouth! My first thought was 'how did a piece of paper get on top of that water bottle spout'. Then I tasted the awful taste and felt this burning sensation on my tongue. I spit out the crackling 'piece of paper' onto my hand. OH my word! It was a stink bug!!!! I ran to the sink and kept shoveling water into my mouth and washing my mouth out. I got a big glass of water and inserted my tongue into the water. It was horrible! The bad taste was gone but the burning sensation was still there! My husband (ex) was concerned at first, but then started to laugh hysterically when he heard about what had happened and saw my utter revulsion and over the top dramatics. He instructed me to drink milk. I did it. Fat free of course (and yes I counted my calories and/or points). I stuck my tongue in that milk and drank it. I don't really like milk, so this in itself was very out of the ordinary for me. Sadly, the milk didn't help. Nothing I did helped! I just had to deal with that nastiness for the next hour or two until it naturally wore off!

The Death

Sixty-four ounces of water is a lot of water! Especially when you are used to drinking next to nothing! I was struggling to figure out how to get my water consumption up to where it needed to be. I tried a multitude of different methods. I had one glass that I filled throughout the day, but I kept losing track of how many glasses I had already drank!   I tried water bottles but that had its issues, mainly that I felt horrible about all of that plastic going into the landfills. I was on a mission to figure this out and find the perfect solution!   I was constantly on the lookout for that perfect solution to arrive in my life. Then, I found it!

I found a water mug that held 64 ounces. This mug was awesome. This mug was double walled giving it a nice insulation so that my water stayed cold yet never left a ring of condensation behind. The mug was clear so I could easily glance at my water to see where I was in my daily drinking adventures for the day. One side of the mug had facts about water and how water was so good for our bodies and the other side had measurement to show exactly how many ounces of water you had left to drink. It was just what I needed. It was perfect for me. I immediately started to use it! I carried that mug with me everywhere. Sure, it was big! It was so big that I referred to it as my water bucket! However, that did not stop me! I carried that water container with me everywhere I went! I took it to work. I took it to family dinners. I even took it into restaurants where I sat my big mug down beside my plate. This water 'bucket' was by my side constantly. I did not just carry the mug. I drank from this mug, constantly! I was drinking so much that I was refilling it halfway through the day! I loved it and it was working for me!

Every day when I left the house, I would carry out my water jug with me to the car. Typically, I was able to immediately place the water on the passenger seat where it rode with me and I would drive away. However, sometimes I would have to juggle things around with where I was putting my water and with anything else that I was carrying. The day of the death was one of those days. I had my hands full and the passenger seat was going to be unavailable as there would be someone riding there. No problem. I moved to the car and placed my water jug on top of the car so that I could finagle my belongings into the backseat before placing the jug on the floorboard by my foot. No problem. I had done this dance a gazillion times with my favorite water jug.   Easy peasy! It was was done. I hopped into the car and off we went.

I had driven about a half mile down the road before I heard a crash. My stomach sank. I knew exactly what it was. I had put the drink on top of the car and hopped in to leave without grabbing my water bucket! The crash could only have been the sound of my water jug flying off the car and hitting the pavement. I reached down to the floorboard, searching and hoping that I was wrong and that my water was in its proper place. Of course, it was not there!

I pulled into the first driveway and made my way back to the scene of the crime. My water jug lay on the pavement in a gazillion pieces! When it hit the ground, it hit in such a way that it shattered. The lid was the only thing that was intact, but that was no consolation. My miracle water jug was history.

I am not kidding you when I said I cried! Literally cried real tears at the death of this water container! It was a very sad day for me!

As a side note, I have spent the last 15 plus years looking for a replacement. I have found similar ones but they are never quite right. I have tried alternative options but they just leave me cold. I have searched high and low for an exact replacement. NOTHING.   It has become somewhat of an obsession as I buy container after container in the quest to get another 'perfect water jug'.   I am hopeful that someday I will once again experience the magic of a perfect water container

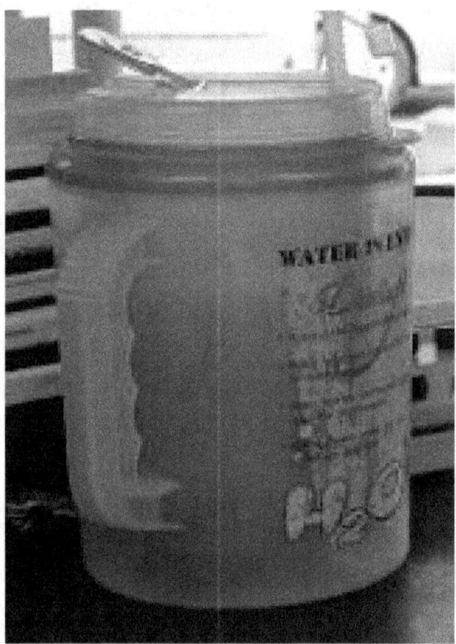

The magical water bucket that I would love to replace!

The switcheroo

I loved my Pepsi. Coke would work too. 7UP, why yes! Mountain Dew was a good choice! I loved my pop (soda). I loved it a whole bunch! I loved it so much that I was drinking insane amounts of it. I am talking 4 or more 20 ounce bottles a day. Water? Who drank that? Certainly not me!   But when I started to look at my health and make changes to actually lose weight and be healthy, I knew that my soda addiction had to change in some way!

I did not want to go cold turkey and go without my beloved drink. That thought was abhorrent to me, at the time. Besides, I was not ready to deal with my caffeine addiction. I decided that I would make the switch from regular full sugar versions of these drinks and move to the diet versions. The only problem? Diet tasted so horrible!   It had the worst aftertaste! However, I was determined. I knew it was something that I had to do!

I made the switch during a week-long vacation from work. I decided that vacation would be the perfect time to make the switch. I knew that we would be traveling and eating out. Furthermore, I knew that I would not be sitting at work staring at a vending machine on each break. I would be away from the habit of drinking multiple bottles during my work day.   I knew that my desire to drink any liquid would be limited to my meals since we would be out sightseeing and visiting friends and family. I just had to navigate the drink situation at each restaurant. I squared my shoulders; I was up for the task.

Oh my word, it was utterly horrible! Each time I would take a drink of my diet soda I could feel my face curl up with distaste. I gagged and made faces. I moaned and groaned. It was not a pleasant experience. I learned to wait until I actually had food in front of me before I actually took a drink. Those first few meals were a catastrophe to my taste buds. It seemed slow, but it really was a fast adjustment. Toward the end of the vacation, I had adjusted to the taste difference and by the time I got home, I was ready to drink only diet soda, even without food to mask the taste!

(Looking back, I know I should have made the leap from soda straight to water. However, I was not at that spot in my life. The switch to water would come later!)

Exercise

I embarked upon a mission to lose weight and I was honestly clueless about what I was doing. At first, I had no real interest in exercise. I was determined to lose weight and never lace up a pair of sneakers. However, I quickly decided that exercise was a great bonus when trying to lose weight.   I operated on the belief that I was only exercising to lose weight for quite a few years. But eventually, I realized that above all else I wanted to be healthy and exercise was instrumental in my quest to be healthy.   I even started to like it a little...sometimes! Exercise brought me some scary moments but it also brought me some moments of laughter as the unexpected was certain to happen to me.

Fool me once.....

My bike was new, Todd and I were running errands after a nice bike ride. The bikes were on the top of the car and we were happy and content. We decided to stop at the local coffee shop. With my infinite wisdom, I decided to go through the drive through window. Obviously, I was forgetting about the bikes that were sitting in the roof rack on the top of my car. I made it into the drive through no problem. However, the problems began when I tried to pull out of the drive through. Crash! I hit the overhead light; totally breaking it and twisting my bike up. The handlebars were facing sideways while the wheels remained straight. Luckily for me, the bike was easily repaired, but I vowed to never do anything so stupid again.

Fast forward two years. It was an exciting day as Todd had just bought a new bike. It was also a gorgeous day outside, perfect for a bike ride. We had a doctor's appointment in the morning and immediately following the doctors visit we purchased his bike. We rushed home to pick up my bike and head out for a ride. "One stop," I said as I drove toward the canal. I swung the car into the pharmacy and up to the pick-up window. Imagine my shock, embarrassment and concern when I pulled in. You see, they have a drive through window with a nice, apparently low hanging sign. You guessed it, Todd's new bike. Yes, the bike that he hadn't even had a chance to ride yet had just smacked into the sign!   Let me tell you, I had some TENSE moments until I realized that his bike was not damaged at all. WHEW!

One more year passed. I was now working at a deli in Sharpsburg, Maryland. One day, a young-looking guy walked in and asked if there was a hotel, or a cab or something. He was looking for anything. He was desperate. My coworker and I quickly set about helping him. We ascertained that he had been trying to ride the whole Chesapeake and Ohio Canal (a National Park that was close by). He had gotten as far as Sharpsburg and was ready to call it quits. He just wanted to go home. He desperately wanted to get on a bus to get there. We quickly devised a plan to get him to a bus station that was about 10 miles away. The problem, he had a bike that he needed to ditch. He was absolutely done and wanted nothing to do with the bike. I decided to take it for parts. I went outside and threw the bike on my bike rack. I didn't have time to lock or secure it tightly at that point since I was at work. So, it was just sitting atop the car. No problem! After work, I was ready to call it a day and get home. I hopped in the car and tore off down the street. I was down to the corner and ready to make a left-hand turn when I remembered that I had just sat the bike on top of the car. I had not secured the bike in ANY way! I made it halfway around the corner when that dang bike FLEW off my car! I was so embarrassed. For a split second I thought about leaving the bike lay where it was and driving away. But reality and responsibility won out. I stopped my car. Vehicles pulled up behind me and blocked traffic. (Luckily for me the bike didn't hit any car or person). The guy from the house at the corner ran out. I just wanted to sink into the ground with embarrassment!   I got the bike back up on the car. This time I properly secured it!   The car sustained one little scratch....and the bike's only damage was a busted chain. That little accident could have been a whole lot worse!

I'm hoping that my stupid bike errors are all behind me!

Self-Sacrificing Sister

When I was about age 12 my family moved from Pennsylvania to Florida. Right before we moved, I had been riding my bike constantly and I had reached the point where my knees were knocking on the handle bars of my hand me down Schwinn bicycle. Therefore, my much-loved banana seat Schwinn didn't travel to Florida with us. I would be getting my very first bike that was purchased just for me. No more hand-me-down bikes! My parents bought me a ten-speed red bike (Schwinn again...because that was THE name in bikes when I was young.) I rode that bike about 2-3 times. Seriously, it's hot in Florida. The pool had more of a draw then riding up and down the road pretending that I was part of the fictional TV show, Chips; like I had done as a youngster. (Ok, maybe budding maturity played a part also.)

Over the next few years my bike collected dust while I rapidly gained weight. However, there was one more occasion where I rode that bike. It was a disastrous occasion! One year while we lived in Florida, my brother got the hair-brained idea that he was going to ride a bicycle from Florida to Maryland. He was serious about his plan. He purchased a nice road bike and all the gear. Every time we went near a bike shop, we would go in so that he could drool and make purchases to aid in his training rides. He went out riding quite a bit and one day he decided that he would like company. Who better to ask than his baby sister. In a fit of insanity, and being the self-sacrificing sister; I agreed to go with him. I dusted off the, like new 10 speed; and told him I was ready to go. We set out. I admit, it was liberating. I enjoyed the hot breeze that wafted over my face. I felt free as a bird. We went into a neighboring community and rode up and down the roads. I was feeling a bit tired but the bike ride was going smashingly well.

Maybe I shouldn't use the word smashingly........

We headed into the section of the neighboring community that was largely undeveloped. We headed down the road and rounded the corner to come back up the hill. Now let me remind you, this was in Florida. It's relatively flat, so I use the term hill loosely. My brother headed up that small incline lickity-split. Me, well it wasn't as lickity-split. My legs were feeling the burn from all the riding, but I turned to follow him up the road.   My lungs filled and I struggled to get a good breath of air as I climbed that hill. I focused on my brother who far ahead of me and already at the top of the hill that wasn't a hill. I kept peddling. It seemed as if I was getting nowhere. I was pushing with all my might but progress up that mammoth mountain road was just not happening.   I leaned over to rest on the handlebars as I cranked on those peddles. Somehow, I lost my balance and that was all she wrote. I went down.

Now, the story diverges a bit. My brother's rendering of this event is a tad bit different. He claims that he was at the top of that road and turned to see where I was. He claims that I was going so slowly as I pushed up the "tiny incline" (according to him it was barely an incline at all) that there was not enough forward momentum to keep me upright. He claims that I even fell over in slow motion.

I suspect there may be a bit of truth in both of our versions. Regardless of which account is exactly correct, I found myself laying on the ground beside my bike. I was embarrassed! My brother sped back down the road to me as I picked myself up. I remember his concern as I hopped on my bike. And rightfully so. I was bleeding and pretty mangled up. I just wanted to get home. Adrenaline must have kicked in because I had more energy and rode faster (at least I felt like I was riding fast) on the trip home. I vividly remember coming to a major road and my brother trying to caution me to slow down and not take any chances, so I must have been a bit foolhardy, reckless and fast riding. At that juncture in the ride, I looked down and saw blood dripping from my knees the whole way down to my socks. Nothing to do but keep riding. I did eventually make it home. I remember getting tweezers and pulling small pebbles out of my hands and knees. It wasn't pretty. It was also the very last time I ever rode that bike. For years I used this accident as just one more reason why I was not going to exercise. Coincidentally, I kept gaining weight!

(My brother never stopped riding. He still rides MAD miles on his bike each week all these years later!)

Can you?

We had already paid for our tour of the Eisenhower Farm. I was excited, I had always wanted to visit the farm at Christmas. We had some time to kill so we went to the battlefield and made our way to one of the towers. We explored a bit before spying a sign marking a hiking trail. By mutual consent we immediately headed down the closest trial. We didn't stop to think about anything. We didn't think about our footwear. We didn't think about the trail conditions (AKA muddy ground.) We just went.

About 500 feet (if that) down the hill my foot slipped in the mud. I couldn't recover my balance and down I went. I heard something pop as I landed with my leg twisted beneath me. It was a struggle to move enough to get my leg out from under me. I was feeling mad pain in my foot. But eventually, I was standing. I tried to place some weight on my foot, it wouldn't hold any weight. Jason motioned to a nearby stump, but I didn't think I could even make it that far at that moment. I stood clinging to him as I kept all weight from that ankle. In that moment, I was convinced that I had broken my ankle. Weirdly enough, I wasn't concerned with the prospect of getting myself back up the hill. I wasn't even concerned about the ramifications of dealing with a possible broken ankle. All I could think about was to ask, "Can you drive Stick Shift?" At that point Jason and I hadn't been dating for long and while it was obvious that I drove manual transmission his capabilities in that regard, had never been discussed. I had no concern that day other than needing to know if he could easily drive my manual transmission car or if I would be giving him a crash course on driving stick shift. If he didn't know, I would be letting him learn to drive stick shift on the fly in my car as he drove, because there was no way I was driving at that point. Jason later told me that he was SURE we were heading to the hospital!

After a few minutes I attempted to put some weight on my foot and much to my delight, I was able to stand on my foot. It was painful, but it worked! We slowly made our way back up the hill to my car. Not only was my foot hurting, but I was covered in mud. Luckily, I had clothes in the car so in the middle of the parking lot (ok, I ducked behind a monument) I changed my clothes. I also switched out of my tennis shoes and put on my hiking boots. I did that for two reasons. I was determined to conquer that hill but I also know that my ankle would fare better with the support of the boot laced tightly around the foot and ankle.   I lamented a bit about the fact that had I been in my hiking boots I probably wouldn't have been hurt. However, hindsight is 20-20.

Being stubborn, we carried on with our day. I actually did conquer that trail.   I also made it to the Christmas at the Eisenhower Farm (what a disappointment....only one room had any Christmas stuff in it and that was a tree and some poinsettias). I also made it to my family Christmas that evening. I did NOT take off my boot until I was home for the evening. I knew the tight lacing would help keep the swelling and pain at bay. I also knew that once the boot was off that it would not be going back on too easily.

Game On

We talked about running every so often. I always talked about getting back to a more consistent training schedule and Jason talked about getting back to running after a long hiatus. His friend and coworker ran long events and eventually Jason broached the subject of us running in one. (The JFK 50 miler to be exact.) I agreed to it, if I was properly trained. We talked, yet neither one of us picked up our feet to go out and run. The

JFK continued to pop up in the conversation for a few weeks but it all was all talk, until one day.

In the midst of all this talk about running it came up that the Donut Alley Rally was a run that I had done for the previous three years, a simple 5K. When Jason heard that the run was scheduled for his birthday that particular year, he was determined to participate! Somehow, in the midst of talking and making our plans, we decided to make running a competitive sport. Basically, it was a competition between the two of us. We would have a weekly competition to see who could run the most miles. We were both all in! The smack talk started almost immediately. And admittedly, I led the charge in the smack talk!

I had seen a spark of competitive spirit a few months previously as we checked out a hotel fitness center. On that day we each hopped on side-by-side treadmills and casually worked our tail ends off to reach that mile mark first. An unwritten competition. It didn't matter that we were only wearing socks and no shoes. It didn't matter that there was no grand prize for the winner. The game was on!

So even with that wee little hint, I was unprepared for the competitive streak that burned strong within Jason. I did laugh that my edge would be in the first few weeks as he got into running shape as I was already conditioned and capable of running 3-5 miles at once. I clearly knew that once he was running consistently that he would run fast and longer than me. I knew this but I planned on enjoying the first few weeks of wins before he took off. I knew this, yet I kept up with a steady stream of smack talk (And yes, we planned on changing the rules as we went along to make this a fair competition.)

Day one of the first week of our competition rolled around. I don't typically run on Mondays, due to my work schedule. My lack of running apparently didn't slow down Jason. I was at work when the running app dinged to notify me of his run. Eagerly I pulled up the app on my phone to view the stats for his first run. The first thing my eyes fell upon was his average pace. Really?? I struggle when I run and I tend to run slow. Jason on his first run, ran at a pace that was easily two to two and a half minutes faster than the average pace that I had most recently run. I then looked at the mileage. 2.46 miles! On his first run in ages! My jaw dropped to my chin. I was blown away. This man just tilted my view of this competition on its axis and it had only just begun.

I retaliated the next morning with a 4.17 mile run. I admit, when I was done, I felt a bit smug with my mileage. I felt good until the next day when Jason's next run popped onto my phone. This time I was in such shock that not only did my jaw drop, but my phone clattered to the desk in front of me. I couldn't believe it! Seriously, I was in shock. It may have even been a bit of awe. Why? This man that I had fallen in love with had posted a 5.22 mile run. FIVE POINT TWO TWO MILES! Oh, and if that wasn't enough, he did it with an average pace of 11 minutes! On his second run. What kind of machine was I dating??? I wasn't down for the count yet! On Thursday I put on my running shoes and went out to run. 6.19 miles! Take that love boy! If I was going to lose, it was not going to be by a landslide! No way!

My 6.19 miles was enough for the win. Jason had pushed too hard too fast and needed to give his aching shin a rest. I was the winner of week one!

Week two started much the same as week one. I couldn't easily run on Monday which allowed Jason to pull ahead in the competition. Yes, he ran 2.02 miles on Monday (once again fast in comparison to me). On Tuesday I went out and ran 2.29, enough to put me in the lead by roughly a quarter of a mile. I ran again on Wednesday.

On Thursday, I got notification of his next run. 2.76 miles. I did the calculations. Woo hoo!! I was still ahead by about a half mile. I texted him to gloat about still being in the lead. He immediately wrote back. "WHAT?" I began to wonder if I had written down a number incorrectly so I popped back into the fitness tracker to check my figures. That is when I saw it. A new run had popped up. This one for one mile. I saw it at the same time that his text came in telling me to, "Check again sweetheart, I ran an extra mile." I couldn't help myself. I busted out laughing. LOUD laughter!

I had gloated too soon. You see he ran 2.76 miles which is when I saw that I was still ahead. Unbeknownst to me, while I was calculating the standings, he had realized the same thing and decided to run an extra mile. That extra mile put him firmly in the lead.

No fears, Friday I got out there and ran 4.47 miles. That meant that on Saturday morning before we met up to spend the day together, he would only have to run 3.88 miles. Was it enough to hold me? I didn't think so...but I was hopeful! Luckily for me, his sister came into town and he spent the morning with his family. Thus, I won again!

The awesome part about winning these weeks? I was able to pick my reward. I choose something outlandish and crazy. I choose something cringe worthy! I chose it not because I wanted it, but because I wanted to watch him squirm! He was so sure that he was going to win that he agreed to my outlandish terms, both weeks! While he and I both knew I would never demand payment for my winnings, I don't think he realized the hold my winnings would have over the upcoming years. You see, even now, almost 10 years later, I will still laughingly bring up my winnings and talk about how "maybe, just maybe it's time for him to pay up."

The Wind Tunnel

I took a ride on the Chesapeake and Ohio Canal. We rode a total of 20 miles that day. Most of the ride was splendid. But the last 2 miles something terrible happened. The last few miles of our ride took us into an open area. We were no longer buffeted by trees.   That was the moment the wind picked up and started to howl. It was terrible. I was in the lowest gear possible and pushing with all my might. My speedometer was only registering that I was going between 1 and 2 mph! All I could do was keep pedaling. While I was pedaling, I was letting out a primal yell from the sheer and absolute horror of the experience. The wind was constant and wouldn't give up.   But even worse, were the occasional gusts of wind that would hit us front and center. The wind was stronger than the pressure that I was exerting to push myself forward and the bike would stop dead in the wind. My speedometer was literally registering as no movement. I swear each time that I would be slightly pushed back. It was brutal.

Girls With Gears

I had reached my doctor approved weight goal and life was looking good. I started to think about how I was going to maintain my weight and keep my motivation high as I continued with this new healthy lifestyle. I looked deep and realized that the one exercise that I truly like to do at that point was to ride my bike. That spurred me to think about participating in some of these bike rides that are out there raising money for nonprofits. I may have mentioned it in my online journal but didn't really make any concrete plans. I just made the decision that it would be a good way to stay motivated. And then one day, I read my online friend Donna's journal. She was setting a goal to do 2 bike rides that year. It got me to thinking and possibly riding in these events with her. I contacted her to get information about the ride that she was first planning on participating in. I got super excited about the event. I asked if she would mind if I tagged along. She welcomed me with open arms. I had roughly 8-10 weeks to prepare to ride 25 miles. I had been riding the recumbent exercise bike, but I knew from experience that the recumbent uses different muscles than an upright bike. I also knew that even when I was riding outside, I rode mainly on the Chesapeake and Ohio Canal, which is flat. That would not work for me as the bike rid that I was signing up for was listed as rolling hills. I knew that I had my work cut out for me. It was still late January or early February, so we quickly got an exercise bike from a friend and it became an integral part of my living room. I rode every day. Six days a week I rode. The bare minimum I rode on those days was an hour. I rode an average of 8-10 hours a week. I rode outside when my work schedule and the weather collided to give me perfect conditions. The perfect conditions for me were sunny and a temperature of about 42 degrees or above. I quickly learned how to dress to stay warm. Determined, I started pushing up and down hills on the road as often as I could.

I rode and rode and rode my bikes in preparation. I figured out that the bike seat on my exercise bike rubbed me the wrong way and I developed a bit of a saddle sore. It hurt, but in a weird way I was proud of my saddle sore. After all, this was a sports injury. Me, Mary Fran having a sports injury, Are you serious????? WOW!

The weather luckily cooperated for me to ride outside at least once each week while I was training for this ride and I hoped and prayed that it was satisfactory to train me to ride 25 miles the day of the event. Exactly 1 month before the event I woke up with a stiff lower back. I knew it would work itself out if I moved it so I jumped on my bike and headed out on the road. I rode and enjoyed my ride and I was right, my lower back pain eased up and totally disappeared. The problem came when I started noticing a pain in my upper back, across my shoulder blade area. I didn't think too much of this, as I've had problems with that muscle in the past. I continued on with life and training. The pain was an ache with a sharp shooting pain occurring every once in a while. It was totally manageable. I wasn't worried. A week went by and it didn't clear up. Two weeks went by and I began to notice that the pain was getting worse. Three weeks and the pain were utter agony and pretty much constant. Everyone was concerned and flipping out. I vowed and promised to go to the doctor AFTER the ride. I was afraid that they would tell me not to ride and I wanted to ride in this event! Then I had the bright idea to visit a massage therapist. I went and found out that my muscle had frozen or seized up. It was going to take many visits to clear up the problem. LOVELY. Being stubborn, I still planned to ride! I had worked to hard to walk away from the event.

This ride, the Girls with Gears was a ride to help raise money for the organization Carol For Heart, which helps educate women and promote awareness that heart disease is the number one cause of death amongst women. I paid my entry fee and even though raising money was not required, I decided to go for it. I'll admit that I wanted to get to the $250 level simply to get the free Bike Jersey. Not to mention that every $25 I raised gave me three raffle tickets for the drawing for a new trek bike! I sent out my email. And I was shocked because the money started to pour in. I made the $250 goal...and the money kept coming. It started to slow down about $400 but it didn't let up. The day before I left to go to my ride, I had raised $490 dollars. I decided to make it an even $500 and put in $10 from my own wallet.

The weekend finally arrived. I was trained. I had raised my money. I was packed and ready to travel the 3 hours to the event. The first stop when I got there was the Spring Mountain Ski Area. It was here that they were holding a mountain bike expo where the Girls with Gears/Carol for heart organization would have a table for early check in for the ride. The plan was to get to the early check in area for the bike event at around 10 or 10:30 and then have the day to sightsee and relax. I was practically giddy to get the swag bag and my long sleeve tee shirt, both of which came with my registration fee. I handed in my money donations and they verified that it was indeed $500. They asked me my size and I soon had my bike jersey in my hand!!!! They then handed me a stack of tickets to submit for the bike drawing. I put my address labels on the stubs (an idea given to me by Donna my bike buddy for this event) and put them in for the drawing.

The race day dawned early. I awoke nervous. I had not been on my actual outdoor bike in exactly 2 weeks! My shoulder had been giving me grief for the last four weeks. Could I do it???? Today was the day. This was it! It was time to sink or swim! I showered and got ready to go. We had breakfast and we were off. We arrived at the park where the ride was to begin at around 7AM. We unloaded our bikes and had a bit of a panic as somewhere and somehow; I had misplaced my bib number. Yes, I know that I was rider number 68...but where was the pesky bib number. I tore apart the bags in the trunk...I searched the car high and low; it was not there! YIKES! Oh well, Donna and I had walked to get the cue sheets and I had figured out that I didn't really need the number as I had already received my goody bag and my meal ticket was actually an armband. Luckily for me, I did have the armband/meal ticket. By about 7:20, we were on our bikes and heading out. We had decided to head out as early as possible so that we didn't have to worry about our speed and we could go at our own pace and stop when we wanted. The scenery was wonderful! The temperature (for the whole weekend) was fabulous! We rode. My head was on a swivel and I babbled on for the first half of the trip. I didn't talk as much the second half. The first half, while hillier was my favorite. We were on back roads. We were basically alone and the scenery was just spectacular!   The second half of the ride was in more developed areas and my body was starting to feel the exertion. I'm sure the choice of my favorite part of this ride was just my personal preference, but I know Donna liked the first half also. I am proud to say that I rode every inch of the ride...which actually ended up being 26 miles instead of 25. I didn't break any speed records and the hills were done at a snail's pace. But I did them!

Getting back to the start/finish line was extremely exhilarating! I had done it! It felt great! We talked a while and then we got in line for our lunch. Lunch for me was a grilled chicken sandwich and a Ceasar salad. (Catered by Outback Steakhouse,) Food tastes so good after exercise. While waiting in line for our food I received the shock of my life. Posted nearby was a list of the top three fundraisers. Whatdaya know? I was number three! While we were eating, I heard them calling my name. I went and they gave me a $100 gift certificate to thank me for my fundraising. It was to the local bike shop! We talked to Andy and Donna for a bit more and then we headed out. We had a long drive home ahead of us and we now had to stop at the bike shop so that I could spend my money. (Oh yeah, and the massage...I paid for a massage on my shoulder before we left the bike event.) At the bike shop I briefly contemplated buying a new bike (I wanted one!) but decided that buying a bike 4 hours from home would not be the most prudent thing. Instead, I bought the cutest bike skort and bike jersey that matched! Absolutely adorable! And then it was off toward home!

My shoulder. I was so nervous about this ride due to my shoulder. I kept praying for my shoulder to be ok for the ride. On Saturday, my shoulder did pretty good. Sunday, the day of the ride; while I could feel a dull ache, the shoulder was GREAT! After my ride I utilized the massage therapists that they had on the premises. It was a dollar a minute donation for a massage. The money would also go toward the organization that put on the ride. I figured it was wise to try to keep my muscle as limber as possible, and the massage therapist from home agreed that if I could get a massage on Sunday to go for it. So, I did. This therapist (the Sunday one) told me that in terms of degree of how bad this is.... on a scale of 1 to 10, with 10 being the worst my shoulder was an 8 at that time. And that was with no sharp pains...only the dull ache. Heavens, what was it before the first massage? I spent much of my time on Saturday and Sunday forcing myself to relax and trying to help my muscles relax. It worked, I completed the ride!

That was the first day that I met Donna (and her Husband Andy). While we had been friends online, that was the weekend that we became friends in real life. We went on to ride in two more bike events that year. Even though we haven't ridden in a bike event together in years, the friendship has continued and is something I treasure greatly.

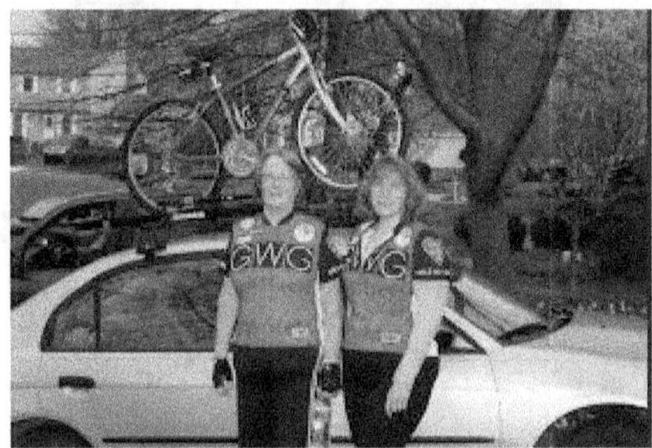

Hiking with Snakes

It was a hot humid summer day. Jason and I were down in the Front Royal, Virginia area for the weekend. We planned to do a shorter hike of no more than four or five miles and then go back to the hotel to swim at the hotel pool. A perfect plan! We decided on hiking to Buzzard Rocks which is in the George Washington National Forest. We set off! We were almost to the top when it happened!

From here the story may diverge depending on which of us is telling the story.

MaryFran's Version:

All was going great as we climbed. We talked and totally enjoyed each other's company. We walked along in the normal manner. For us, that is with myself in the front and Jason bringing up the rear. As we moved up the trail, I focused on the natural steps in front of me. (Either a stone or a log.) The next thing I knew, I noticed crazy movement at my feet. I looked down and to my horror I saw a snake slithering across my booted foot! This snake was huge!!! Monstrous in fact!!! And I swear, I saw it wrapping its reptilian body around my ankle! Thank goodness I was wearing a high boot! I screamed. Probably loudly! Luckily the monster snake slithered away and I high tailed it a few feet further up the trail. I was sure this snake had a "partner" nearby! I had barely escaped with my life, but I had made it!

Jason's Version:

We were walking along almost to the top of the trail. We were just enjoying the views and companionship. My attention shifted away from the trail to look at some aspect of nature that had caught my eye. And then I heard the panicked scream from MaryFran. "I thought you had seen a big spider," I later remarked to her, once I knew she was safe. By the time I figured out the problem was a snake, the danger was past. The poor innocent snake was already slithering away and MaryFran was making fast progress in moving away from the area as fast as she could! Immediately, I leaned over to inspect the wee tiny garter snake. It was so cute.

I did go back to get a closer view of the "monstrous" snake. It was definitely not happy as it hissed at me. I guess I scared it as badly as it scared me. I survived!   Jason survived my snake encounter too! And according to Jason as he later said, "It's a good thing, you didn't step on the snake, it would have killed it", so apparently the snake survived also!

You get what you Pay for

I do not know what possessed me to buy a bike. Maybe my choice was due to the influence of my brother who is an avid biker. It could have been simply a whim. Whatever the reason, that is exactly what I did. I bought a bike. I did my research before making my purchase. I did not want to buy a cheap bike. First, my brother probably would have disowned me had I purchased something cheap. Secondly, I had a method to my madness. I know me. I can be a bit cheap (or should I say frugal) and I knew that if I spent hundreds of dollars on a bike that I would feel compelled to actually use the bike.   I researched every component and spent some time discussing with my brother bikes and bike parts. The day finally came and I bought my bike! I was so excited to go out and ride! I called my boyfriend at the time and we headed out to ride.

 My boyfriend at the time decided to buy a bike so that he could ride with me! I was so happy! What is better than riding by yourself? Riding with someone else!   I tried to lay out all of my research and thoughts on bikes to help him with his decision.

He wanted nothing to do with my thoughts and ideas. He marched himself into one of these big box stores and purchased a bike off the rack. Now I have nothing against the big box stores. However, there are some things that you want to make sure that you buy that are high quality. Bikes are one of them and usually the bikes you find in these stores are usually not of any great quality. However, this was his decision. He was actually insistent that his bike that he saved so much money buying was awesome and even better than mine was! It was his money and his choice so I just sat back and let him do his thing.

Off we went riding.   His bike needed to go into a bike shop for a repair within the first two weeks. My bike was running slick as a whistle.   I tried to keep my smug grin to a minimum.   A few weeks later, his bike malfunctioned again. When this second issue cropped up it happened in the middle of a long ride. Luckily, the malfunction did not affect the ability of the bike and was an issue that affect the comfort. I offered to swap bikes periodically so that he could get relief from the discomfort of his bike. That was when I saw the true disadvantage of buying a cheaper bike. The bike was a monster. There was not one ounce of joy in riding that bike. The pedals turned so sluggishly. It was as if they were stuck in quicksand. They had a gritty rough feeling as they spun. The gears did not shift smoothly. The list went on.   Nothing was right with this bike.

Meanwhile, I looked at my boyfriend. The smile on his face as he rode my bike was pure elation. He was feeling the beauty of riding a bike that had decent if not good components. It was night and day different and there was no way that he could pretend that he did not notice the difference. He did not want to give me back my bike!

He got his bike repaired again that time and I did give that bike one more chance. Yes, I got back on that cheap bike and gave it a ride. It was pure misery! He knew that he had made a mistake. As soon as his money allowed, he bought a new bike (ironically enough the same make and model as the bike I was riding at the time). Once he got his new bike, he never again rode that cheap bike.

You actually used it

I decided to buy myself a new bike. This was going to be a large purchase for me and I wanted to do it right.   I did the research. I looked at the components on various bikes. I checked out different bike shops. I did my homework and eventually I settled on a bike and a bike shop. I was so super excited to go in to buy my bike. I was also nervous.

Why was I nervous? I was overweight. I felt self-conscious to go into a bike shop where the people selling the bikes were super fit and lean. I felt way out of my league as I walked into the shop to make my purchase. I had done my due diligence before I went to purchase the bike though, so it did not take me long to make my purchase. Within a short time, I was the owner of a new bike! The sale people were super nice as I made my transaction. They even helped me load the bike onto my new bike rack.   But my discomfort did not abate until I drove away

I wasted no time and headed out for a bike ride.   The first ride was interesting. I was certainly sore. After all, I was seriously overweight. However, it felt amazing!   It was so freeing and liberating! I could not wait to do it again.   I kept riding every chance I could. I could feel myself getting stronger.

My bike came with a complimentary tune up at a predetermined interval after purchase. I had put the tune up on my calendar and when the time came, I dutifully loaded my bike and took it back to the bike shop.   I was a pro as I unloaded the bike from the car's bike rack. After all, I had been loading and unloading my bike every chance I could get. I wheeled my bike in and the first person I saw was a sales person. In fact, the very same sales person sold me my bike.

"Oh my word! You've actually been riding your bike!" He blurted out with excitement. I looked at him, a bit startled at his words. I think he realized exactly how he sounded and he tried to make it better by explaining. "We sell so many bikes and we know that they will never be ridden. I thought yours would be one of those. Look at you! It is super obvious that you've been riding."

Honestly, I do not know if he knew that I was riding from the obvious dirt on my bike or if he actually noticed my burgeoning muscles in my legs. Whatever his reason for his deduction, I was tickled that my hard work has noticed!

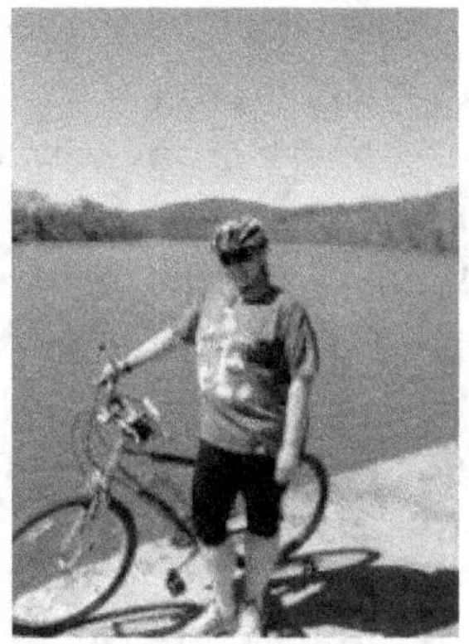

A much used and loved bike.

Freight Train

I had met this really awesome guy and I was super excited! I had been single for a while and had quite frankly just about given up on ever finding a guy to hang out with and do things with. I almost gave up, but then along he came, Jason had come into my life! We had only been dating about a month before we decided to go for a hike. What better than a hike to a waterfall? I was not worried about the hike. I knew that I had never really spent a whole lot of time hiking at that point in my life. However, I knew that I was in decent shape due to the hours of Zumba and the number of miles that I was running each week. The weather was perfect as we left headed down the trail. It was the middle of December but we only needed sweatshirts.

We were hiking in the Shenandoah National Park and the scenery was fabulous. We had a wonderful time as we headed down the trail toward the waterfall. It was a perfect date. We admired the nature that surrounded us, had some nice conversation and we enjoyed each other's company. We eventually reached the waterfall. We spent some time at the top of the waterfall and we were feeling so awesome that we even hiked down to the bottom of the waterfall. It was spectacular! However, eventually we knew that we needed to hike back up the trail and to the car so that we could get home at a relatively decent hour. Off we went.

What goes up must go down! Except in this case, we had gone down the trail on the way to the waterfall. That meant that the return trip to the car was all uphill! We started up the trail and I was quickly feeling as if my lungs were going to explode! I swallowed deeply. This was in the early stages of our relationship and there was no way that I was going to slow down or let on that I was feeling the effects of this hike! No way! I pushed on.

I began to breathe more deeply with the exertion. I was fighting to keep my breaths short and even. I focused intently on my breathing. I did not want to sound like a freight train following him the hill.   I tried to suck air into my heaving lungs as quietly as I could.   On every exhalation I would try to push my exhale through my nose as it was quieter than using my mouth. I was working double time to try to keep my agony a secret. All because I was on a date with a hot guy! I wanted to slow down! I wanted to give up! I wanted to sigh and moan.   I shot a quick glance over at Jason. To my eyes, he seemed to be practically dancing up the hill with no effort.   No way was I letting this handsome man see my agony. I redoubled my efforts. I kept hiking the same pace without a single word of discomfort. I continued to try to draw in air to my screaming lungs without gasping like a dying fish. Trying to be as quiet as possible. I prayed for the trailhead to be around each bend.

I made it off that trail in one piece. I was a sweaty mess and I took comfort in the fact that Jason was also a sweaty drenched mess! I took pride in the fact that I felt as if I had managed to keep my struggle a secret!

Years later Jason and I were talking about that hike and I laughingly said that the biggest thing I remember about that day was my struggle to keep my breathing even and not sound like a freight train. He started to laugh and had to come clean with me. He admitted that he had been breathing heavy himself and did not even notice my struggle!

In retrospect, the trail was definitely an ascent to get back to the car. However, the trail was not that horrid. It was only made difficult due to my mission to keep my freight train breathing a secret. The trail itself was nowhere near the worst that I have hiked. But it is my least favorite type of trail in that it starts with the descent.   I have come to hate trails that start with a descent! I prefer to get the hard part a hike completed first so that when I am already tired from the first part of the hike that I can enjoy the easier descent.

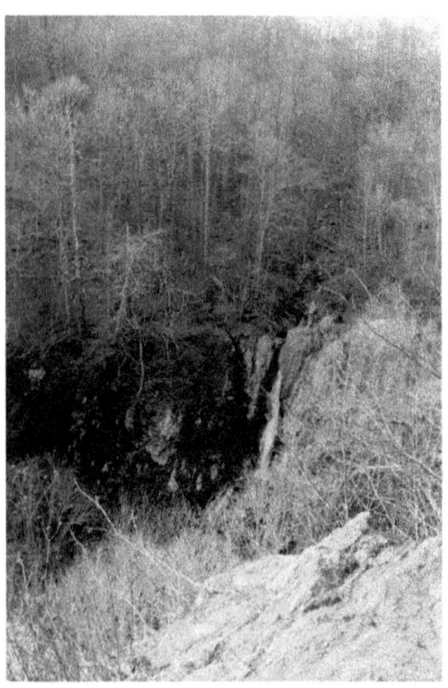

The waterfall we hiked to

Who Knew

I had owned my comfort/hybrid bike for quite a few years and I had actually put a fair number of miles on the bike but I had never really taken it off road. The most 'off road' I had ever gone was the C & O Canal, and that is quite tame. But when Jason bought a mountain bike, I knew that my off-road days were probably just beginning. We talked about my fears of some of those mountain bike trails and hesitantly, I agreed to try out some easy trails.

It took a while but a long weekend away was the time to put action behind my words. The weather was forecasted to be absolutely gorgeous so we carted our bikes to Staunton, VA to enjoy the long weekend.

Jason did his research and found a trail that was labeled as a great beginner/easy trail. There was only one wee slight problem. We couldn't find any address for the trailhead. That address was nowhere online and the visitor center in the town didn't have a clue either! The representative at the visitor center directed us to where she thought it was. So early the next day we headed west from Staunton toward the West Augusta Trail.

Ok, there was another wee problem. We never found the trail! We found Braley Pond though! This is a very pretty little pond with a picnic ground nearby. We were not going to give up, so we decided to strike out on the trail leading from the picnic area at Braley Pond. If it got too difficult, we would turn around, right?

The first half mile to mile was relatively easy and then it got really rocky. Technical rocky too! I was having to focus on where to direct my tires. But I pushed on. I was not a sissy and I was not giving up! We did momentarily think about stopping but as luck would have it a lady walking a dog hiked by and we were able to ask her about the trail up ahead. Her words before she walked off were "It gets much smoother as you get to the hill and when you go down it's pretty easy, just go slow because there is a drop off on one side of the trail." We looked at each other and Jason deferred the decision to myself (the newbie). I was game. Let's go on, I declared!

She was right, the trail did smooth out as we went uphill. And she was right, we reached the top and we started to go down with a drop off to the right. It was liberating to go downhill! I picked up some speed as we started to descent the hill! I was loving it!

And then I realized that I was going a bit too fast. I started to try to slow down.

**Who knew that the bike wouldn't slow down easily on a bed of pine needles?

**Who knew that there would be a big tree root obstructing the trail?

**Who knew that one must keep their feet more parallel midway through the rotation of the peddle while not peddling?

**Who knew that front brakes when going downhill are not the smartest decision?

Yeah, it was a comedy of errors and I went down! Head over the handlebars I went down!

Almost immediately upon doing my face plant on the trail. (Yes, thankfully I didn't fly off the drop off immediately to the right of the trail.) I knew that I was ok. I darted a look back to make sure that Jason was not barreling down the hill to accidentally run me over! He had stopped, but the look on his face was absolute terror and horror! I couldn't help but laugh!

I didn't waste time bemoaning my fall or any possible issues. I picked up my bike and prepared to get back on. I had a trail to finish! I don't know if I was dazed or shook up or what, but as I pointed the bike in the right direction it didn't look right. I asked Jason, "Is my front wheel backwards?" He gently confirmed it (Probably horrified and even more worried about my mental stability at that moment!) and I righted the tire and hoped back on.

I went a whole lot slower this time. I made it to the bottom and completed the trail! Oops, I don't think that was a newbie trail.

Injuries sustained? My wrist was a bit sore and a bit swollen. My elbow was a bit bruised and brush burned. And the inside of my calf had a nasty looking huge bruise within a few hours. All in a day's bike ride.

Jason laughed about his bad ass girlfriend that did an endo on her first trip and got back on the bike.

We did get back on the bikes the next day. We went to Montgomery Hall Park and hit all their trails. The red trail was perfect. Some uphill that was difficult but not too technical for a newbie like myself. The red trail dropped us onto the blue trail and that was absolutely terrifying! I walked over obstacles and just looked in awe at the jumps! I took the blue trail VERY slow! The blue trail ended and we jumped on the yellow trail to make our way back to the car. That was a bit easier than the blue trail...but still rough. But other than having to walk over some of the larger obstacles and up some of the hills, I did it.   In fairness, some of the blue trail could have been myself being timid after my fall the day before!

It wasn't until after we put the bikes on the car and headed home and were talking about the bike ride that Jason figured out that I had no clue how to get over a log other than just hope that if I hit the log fast enough that I would roll over it. Who knew you could pull up on the handle bars and pop over it! Apparently just like popping a wheelie. Who knew? (And who knew how to pop a wheelie....but I have a feeling I'll know soon enough!)

Disc Brakes

It was Labor Day and we had headed up to Canaan Valley in West Virginia for a weekend of biking. Jason had his Santa Cruz and I had my Trek Navigator. The Trek Navigator is a bike that is classified as a comfort bike. It is built for comfort, not for mountain biking. I was worried about navigating the trails on my comfort bike. I knew that I was pushing the bike and myself well past its limits on the mountain bike trails. But I was determined. While we were up roaming around the small town of Davis, West Virginia we walked into the bike shop. The idea was born to rent me a bike. I could rent a bike that would be more capable on the trails that we wanted to ride. We rented a Santa Cruz Chameleon for me and we headed off to Canaan Valley resort to ride some trails that were labeled easy. I eagerly hopped on the rented bike and took a swing around the parking lot before heading off down the trail. It was kind of awkward at first but I was getting used to it and the trail wasn't too difficult at the beginning. We came to a wooden bridge over a marshy area. The entrance onto the bridge was at was at an angle and I panicked and threw on the brakes. Well, what do you know, that puppy had disc brakes! Apparently disc brakes are a tad bit touchier than my old-fashioned brakes on the trusty comfort bike. Or maybe, it was just the fact that the wood on the bridge was a bit wet. Whatever the reason, I went down. I was able to hop back up, laugh and move on with the bike ride.

It was a great workout. While easy, it was still a challenging trail to ride. (Even Jason went down once). I kept repeating a certain phrase in my head during that ride. "Trust the bike." I knew that I had to trust the bike to get me over little twigs and bricks and small obstacles. Things that I normally would not have been able to get over in my comfort bike. I had to trust the bike, trust the tires and trust the suspension.

After our ride I was wiped out!!! I slept like a log that night! The only casualty, other than my pride was the pants I was wearing. During my fall they had gotten chain grease all over the leg.

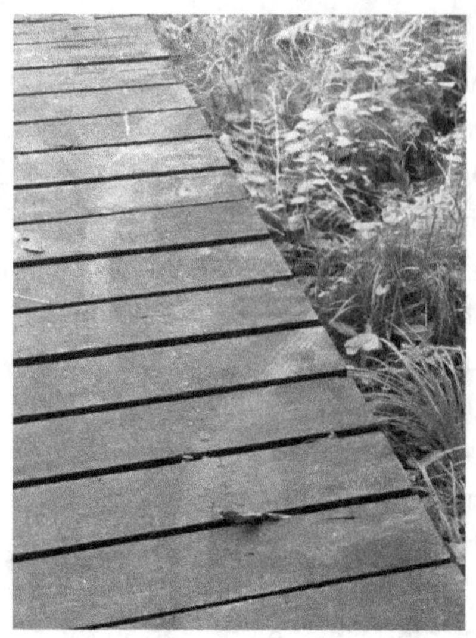

The bridge where it happened, notice the skid marks

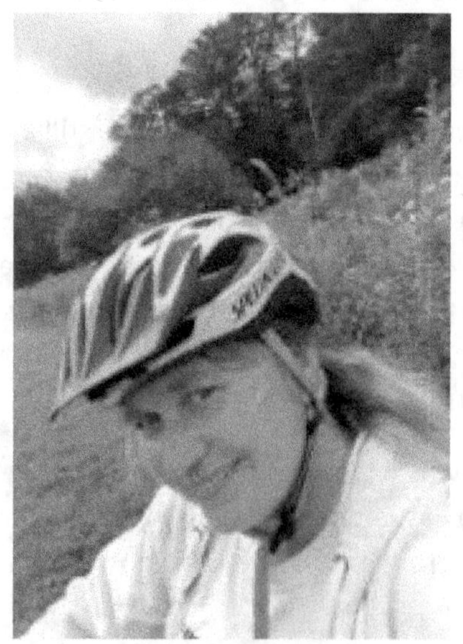

I was still smiling even after my tumble.

First Ride

I finally did it! I replaced my trusty 'comfort' bike with a real mountain bike. (Well, I didn't replace it, the Trek Navigator was an old friend. I kept it!)   For my first Trail ride on my new bike, we decided to head to Little Bennett Park Regional Park in Maryland and ride the same trail that I had ridden a few months previously on a different bike. I figured that if I could handle that trail on a bike that was not made for the trail then I could definitely handle it on a bike that was made for the trail. It was hot but that did not deter us as we set off. I started down the trail. Immediately, I felt out of control. I felt like I was going to fly off the bike. Every turn/corner made my breathe catch. I decided to slow it down a bit. I turned my head so that I could talk to Jason who was following behind me.

"Which breaks do I want, "I questioned? "The right or the left?" I was not joking. I was dead serious; I truly didn't know and I needed the answer! I didn't want a repeat of the flip over the handlebars that I had previously had. I had learned my lesson! I just needed a little review of how to avoid that fate! With my question answered I safely slowed down my bike. Going slower made me feel less out of control and while I wasn't exactly enjoying myself. I wasn't miserable. I might not have been miserable, but I was terrified! I didn't know how my bike was handling around the curves and I didn't know what to expect when I hit a bump. It was just a new experience. I was still very tentative as we went down large hills. But I was starting to feel more and more confident with each rotation of the petals.

We got to the end of the trail and decided to ride down the fire road (all downhill...fun!!). We got to the bottom and headed down the next trail/road. We went across a bridge and came to the mud pit. I saw an opening in the grass to the side of the trail so I headed in that direction and came up upon a small obstacle, a root. And I lost my balance. I teetered toward the puddle. I was sure I was going to go head first into the mud!!!! I saw my 'life flash before my eyes'. Ok, that's a bit dramatic, but I could see myself covered from head to toe in mud for the rest of the ride and the drive home. Somehow, I saved it though and didn't go down!!! I did however smack my calf hard against the peddle!

We got to a point in our ride where we were really hot and thirsty. And that is when we realized that neither one of us had brought water along. I had always been the one to carry the water in my water cages on my old bike and in the extra saddlebags that I had on that bike. I had chosen to not put water cages on the new bike. I knew that I would be buying a hydration pack within a few weeks. Unfortunately for us, that time hadn't come yet and I didn't even think about grabbing the water from the car. No other option was available to us. It was time to turn around and make our way back to the car. We vowed to just find another trail should we feel like ridding more after we got our water, which was in the car. We rode to the bottom of the fire Road and we headed up the hill.

My hill climbing abilities are really weak. But I was determined. My brother's words came back to me. I put the gear into the easiest one possible and I started peddling with all my might. I kept going up that hill fully expecting to have to stop at any moment. Somehow, I made up that hill without my feet touching the ground once. I took a breather at the trail head and that is where I knew what my personal challenge was going to be.

I didn't tell Jason what my challenge was going to be. I just set off on the trail. My personal challenge was that I was determined to ride that trail without stopping. That trail was mostly uphill and I was determined that I was not putting my feet down. Very early on I was starting to breathe like a freight train. I focused on my breathing and tried to count my breaths to regulate myself. But my feet didn't touch the ground on the first uphill section. I reached a flat section of the trail, maybe even a slight downhill. I breathed a sigh of relief anxious to catch my breath. But the uphill came right back. Along with the uphill, came legs that were aching and burning. That was coupled with breathing that became even more choppy and harsh. Still, my feet did not leave the peddles. I pushed forward. I was slow, I'm sure. But I kept pushing through the pain and the ragged breaths. At one point I remember muttering a prayer, "Dear God let this trail end!" I came to a feature on the trail that I recognized and I knew that I was getting close to the end.   Closer but not there yet.

It must have been very apparent that I was really pushing hard and struggling. I heard Jason make a comment to me from behind me. "It's not worth hurting yourself over." He had not been told what my mission was, but he recognized it nonetheless. I think he was concerned.

I kept getting closer to the end of the trail. It was going slowly, at a crawl it seemed! I began to dream about how I would be able to get off the bike and sit down beside the car. I imagined how the grass would feel as I lay down. I knew that my tires were going to leave the dirt trail and I was stopping immediately. I couldn't wait! I pushed on toward the end.

I made it! I got my tires off of that trail, I sat down and immediately leaned against the trail head marker. I had done it! It wasn't pretty. It wasn't fast. It was in no way graceful. But there the sense of pride and accomplishment that overcame me. I struggled to not cry. I was euphoric with satisfaction. Jason brought me a nice cold water. That was the best water! I had him take a picture of me. It's not that often that my sense of pride is quite so strong.

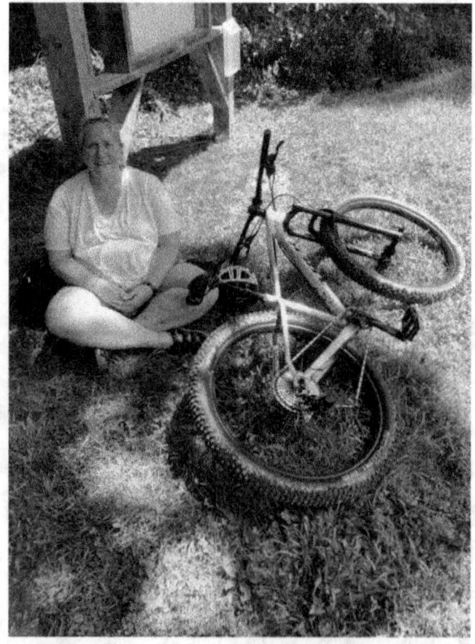

I was so proud of myself!

Trail of Tears

Ready or not, it was time. I had finally agreed to go for a mountain bike ride on a trail that Jason and I had hiked.   Since we had hiked the trail, I knew that the trail was a flow trail, meaning that the trail was smoother and did not have many difficult features to navigate through or across. Jason knew that even though I was new to mountain biking that I would be capable of riding the trail. I was the one that was not certain about my capabilities. The trail was long. The trail was not flat or downhill, it was …. well a flowy trail that had uphill sections followed by downhill sections. I knew I had the downhill sections in the bag. I love to go downhill and I love to go fast. It was the uphill sections and the length of the trail that had me concerned. I had not built up any great endurance nor were my hill climbing skills up to snuff. Therefore, I was quite worried. However, I did not say no. Off we went to the trail!

It was a gorgeous fall day. The air had just a touch of crispness and the leaves were starting to fall. We headed down the trail. That mountain bike trail actually started with a short incline and then began a windy low-grade descent. I struggled up the incline. It was not an easy start to our ride but then we started to go down that windy descent. I absolutely killed the downhill portion. It was fun. But what goes down must go up. The trail began to twist and climb a bit. I was breathing hard. I was struggling but I was doing it…mostly. I would push myself up the inclines by sheer will power and then I would relax and enjoy the decent. However, each time we hit a hill it became harder and harder for me to complete. Finally, my body and mind had enough and I stopped. I am sure Jason expected me to take a breather and either get back on the bike and finish the hill or at the very least walk up the hill. What he got was something very different. I pulled my bike off the trail and I plopped myself down into a pile of leaves and immediately burst into tears.   The epitome of patient, Jason encouraged me and talked me through my upset. The bike ride was over, as much as it can be when you are two miles from the car.

On the way back to the car I did the best I could. I alternately rode and walked that bike back to the car. Boy was I ever glad to see the car!   Once I was safe at home, we talked about it and dubbed the trail the "trail of tears" as I had obviously christened the trail with my tears.

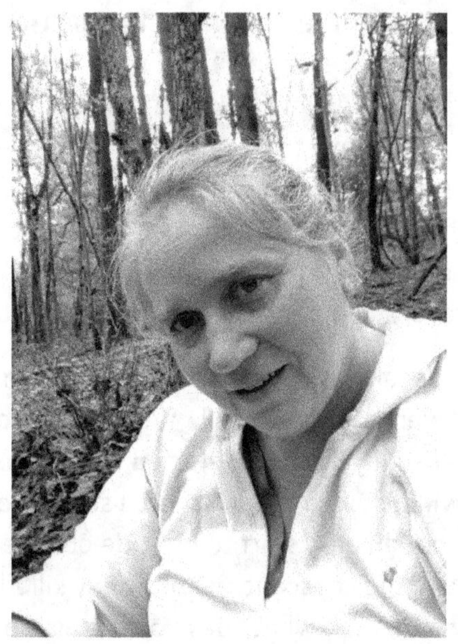

Jason was in such shock at my actions that he snapped a picture of me sitting along the trail.

Trail of Tears Redux

After our brief experience on the trail of tears Jason was more excited to back out there and try it again. He had enjoyed the super flowy trail and was actually disappointed that he hadn't had the chance to complete the whole trail.   Me on the other hand wanted to avoid it at all costs. It had not been a pleasant experience for me at all.   I had not given up on mountain biking. I just steadfastly had been refusing to go to the trail of tears. We went to a different regional park where I was having a blast, and getting better each time we went out on our mountain bikes. I was content with the thought of never having to ride the 'trail of tears' again. However, Jason never forgot. He was patient and waited for me to gain some confidence and a little more endurance before he started to encourage me to go back to my nemesis. He talked the trail up and even refused to use my name for this demon trail and insisted on calling the mountain bike trail by its real name. I wanted nothing to do with that trail and I held off as long as I could. In fact, it was well into the next summer before he was able to talk me into attempting this trail again.

I finally agreed to give it a try so we geared up and headed out. I actually handled the first incline smoothly. I was still pushing hard to complete it, but I made it without any fear of falling off due to pedaling so slowly. (Which of course has sadly happened to me in the past.) Maybe I could do this! Jason called out encouragement as we rode and I kept riding. We made it through the first decent and then back up the next hill. Up and down we went. We passed the spot where I had stopped and cried during my first attempt at the trail of tears. I was feeling tired, but I kept pushing that bike forward. We crossed a stream and then another one. I was doing it but I was so tired. I began to hurt more and more. However, I didn't want to stop because Jason was having so much fun and I didn't want to ruin his good time. So, I soldiered on. In my head, one phrase kept repeating itself over and over. This isn't fun. Over and over again, it repeated in my head. This isn't fun. This isn't fun. This isn't fun.

I refused to stop. I kept pedaling that mountain bike up hills and down hills. All the while that mantra, "This isn't fun" was beating a steady rhythm in my head. Before long silent tears joined the phrase that was pounding in my head. Yet I still continued on. It wasn't until we came to a longer climb that I reached my breaking point. I saw the climb ahead of me and I started to pedal my mountain bike up that hill. By this time great gulping sobs of self pity had arrived.   In case you don't know, sobbing and exercise is not exactly a good match. Half way up the hill I had had enough. I stopped dead in the middle of the trail. I climbed off that cursed bike and dropped it right where I stopped and I sat down where I proceeded to give in to the urge to have a good cry.

Luckily, Jason had the presence of mind to quickly realize that I had stopped the bike on hill right before a blind turn. "You can't just stop there; someone is going to get hurt!" He exclaimed! Any bike coming down the hill would have slammed into me and my abandoned bike, most likely causing damage to everyone involved.   His first order of business was to get me off the trail. He helped me to stand and helped me off the trail and to a safer place to sit.   He then hastened back to the trail to retrieve my abandoned bike.

Even as he was ensuring our safety, he was soothingly saying over and over. "It's over. We are done." He was so distraught over my tears that I didn't have the heart to scream out what I really wanted to say which was "It's not over, I still have to ride about 5 miles back to the car."   Jason was the epitome of patience with me that day. He sat and encouraged me while I sobbed on the side of the trail. He rode beside me on the way back and didn't say a word about my slow pace. And yes, I did ride my mountain bike out of those woods that day. I even had enough energy to wipe my tear stained face and ride like the wind whenever we would come up on people hiking. My pride

was still intact and I didn't want to let anyone else see me
struggle!

After this second experience on this horrid mountain bike trail,
Jason threw up his hands and began calling it the trail of tears
also.   It had proven itself worthy of the name!

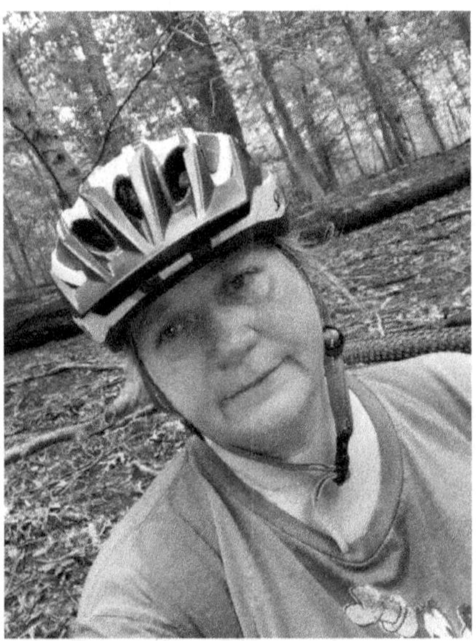

I didn't even have it in me that day to wipe my tears for the picture.

The trail of Tears Onward

And still, Jason never gave up on the idea of riding the complete
length of the trail of tears. He wanted to complete that full trail
like nothing else. It was only a week or two after my second
crying jag on the trail that he started to push to ride it again. He
had complete confidence in my abilities and saw the ability
within myself. He also recognized what I would not admit out
loud, and that was that my failure was all due to the voices in

my head that said that I couldn't do it and that it wasn't fun. Those voices had gotten louder and louder until I could no longer ignore them. I had given up not due to any physical restriction but rather a mental one. He brought up the possibility of another try on the trail of tears. I steadfastly refused and pushed instead to ride in my safe haven park and the bike trails there. But it was only a week or two later before we were back at the trailhead for the "trail of Tears". This time, I rode past the first crying hole. I powered past the hill where I had been emotionally broken and thrown the bike down in a fit of tears. I pushed onward and I made it to the end of the trail. I had completed it and I felt amazing. Tired, but amazing. I even made it the whole way back to the car without any tears. (The Trail of tears is an Out and back trail.) I had conquered the trail!

I wasn't comfortable with the trail. It was still my nemesis. Jason however, loved that trail. So, I was unable to avoid it. We went back to the trail repeatedly and I actually started to feel more comfortable. I got passed by every bike rider on the trail, but I was out there pushing those pedals round and round. Dare I say I even enjoyed it a bit?   However, the true victory was the day that we parked the car as some mountain bike riders departed from the trailhead. We didn't pay any attention to them. They were ahead of us and would quickly leave us in the dust, just like every other rider had. Since they had a 10-minute head start we were sure that we would only see them when they turned around for the return trip to the car. We got our bikes off the car, threw on our helmets and off we went. It was a nice day for a bike ride. The trail was shaded, it wasn't too hot, and we were both feeling good.   We quickly dispatched the opening incline and the fun descent down to the first stream/bridge crossing. We didn't even pause as we headed up the next incline. We had just made it to the top when something crazy happened. I saw those biker riders right

in front of us.   REALLY? I was going to pass someone! Me???
Surely not!

That is exactly what happened! I came up behind those riders
and used every bit of etiquette that I had learned to safely pass
them. I was polite, but I couldn't keep the huge grin off of my
face! I had done it! That was my first time riding up on and
passing another bike rider on a mountain bike trail! And it
happened on my nemesis trail, the trail of tears. How about
that!

Tenderloin

"Look, I hurt myself," I playfully whined as we got back into the
car after getting Slurpies at 7-Eleven. I had simply pinched my
finger on the machine and given myself a tiny blood blister.   We
inspected my grave injury and I received a "healing kiss" to
make it all better. We laughed and I admitted that I would
whine and joke about stupid injuries but if I were to really be
injured, I would downplay how badly I was hurt and not even
tell anyone if I could get by with keeping it a secret.

Prophetic words for sure! I don't think either of us realized how
soon those words would come back to haunt me! Happily we
headed off to our days destination, Mason Neck, a Virginia State
Park. We were going hiking. The weather was gorgeous! We
started off to hit some of the trails in this gorgeous park. I was
ok at the beginning. But a few miles into the hike I began to feel
a hot spot forming on one heel. We hadn't carried a day pack
with any supplies, so I did the only thing that I could. I
tightened my shoe laces to make them tighter to hopefully

alleviate the issue. By the time we reversed directions to return to the car, both of my heels had hot spots. I quietly adjusted the laces again. The walk back was murder. The hot spots were no longer hot spots but rather blisters the size of Texas. (Yes, I am prone to over exaggeration!) It hurt, but I didn't say a word. Jason later told me that walking behind me, he couldn't even detect a limp or any change in my gait. I kept it a great secret!

When Jason started walking more slowly because of a muscle issue, I was SO relieved! Muscle issue? He was having a muscle in his groin area that was giving him some serious pain. I could tell that he was in pain, but we had no option other than to hike onward. Watching him and worrying about his pain did also help take my mind off the searing pain of the blisters.

I may have mentioned in passing as the evening moved on that I "picked up a blister or two", but I totally downplayed the severity. We spent the evening watching him and trying to ease the cramping and muscle aches of his tender muscle. Admittedly, I got the giggles and did laugh quite a bit because it was in his groin area and the area was tender, making it a tender-loin (like the meat). It was a rough evening for both of us in that regard.   As long as nothing touched my heels, I was fine. As for Jason, it wasn't pretty. He was cramping up really bad and paced the room quite a bit!

The next day we walked at Huntley Meadows, a local park. I had wrapped and tried to protect my blistered feet but it was a painful day. Jason didn't fare any better. His tenderloin was kicking something fierce. About 4 miles into the day and we were done. We drove home and stopped to pick up dinner at Jimmy Johns. We were quite the pair as we hobbled into the restaurant. It was a really painful shuffle! For about a week after this hike I didn't wear any shoe that touched my heel.

Jason did realize how bad these blisters really were at some point and I finally revealed my blisters. However, I didn't reveal the mammoth blisters until after we were done hiking. Oops! I did however give him fair warning that I would downplay any injures. He learned his lesson, the next time we hiked, he visually inspected my feet. He also still frequently asks about my feet, knowing I won't lie if asked outright. Guess that is a lesson learned!

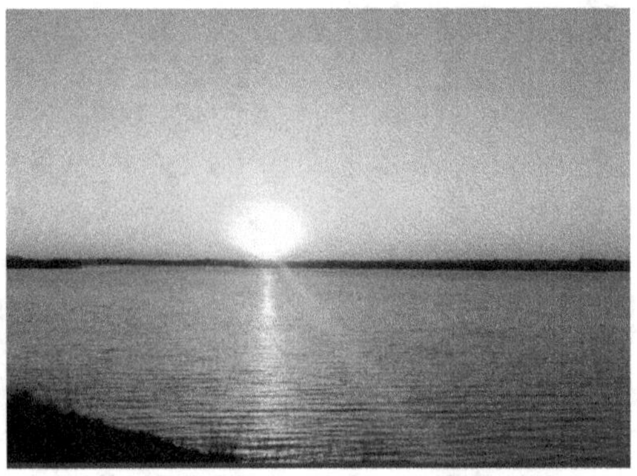
The sunset at Mason's Neck was gorgeous

The Double Stumble

Some of life's scariest moments turn out to be the funniest things. Take for instance a simple walk.

Walking late at night during my college years became a soothing and relaxing habit that I enjoyed frequently with my friend Suzy. We used it as a way to unwind but also to exercise a bit. They do say that exercise is one of the best medicines for stress! It is probably one of the reasons that my time in college marked one of my lowest weights as an adult.

The night in question started simply enough. The air was still a bit cold, but spring was definitely on the way. Suzy and I started out on our walk. Relaxed, we walked down the road toward our dorm, which was about a mile off of campus. We were ready to return to our rooms refreshed. As we talked, we watched the slowly approaching dorm building. Noticing a plume of smoke rising above the building, I grabbed Suzy's arm drawing us both to a complete stop.

Figuring the smoke was coming from somewhere beyond the dorm, we kept our panic in check. To be on the safe side, we decided to walk around the building to find the origin of the smoke.

Veering off the well-lit road, we walked side by side as we entered a narrow dark area in the trees beside the building. Stumbling in a little hole, I paused to regain my balance. This allowed Suzy to move a few paces ahead of me. As I recovered, I followed Suzy. Suddenly, out of the blue I heard Suzy let out a loud screech and watched as she turned on her heel and ran, past me and back to the well-lit road. Not exactly sure what was happening, I continued on the path that Suzy had abandoned. Don't ask me why. I really don't know. Momentary lack of brain power is my excuse.

All of a sudden, I realized, with startling clarity exactly why Suzy had fled the premises!

Standing before me were two guys dressed in black, hiding in the shadows. Unsure of their intent, I turned and started running away. Not sure exactly what was happening behind me, I ran for dear life. I had no idea if these guys were chasing me! And then disaster struck!   As I ran, my foot found the same hole that I had found as I walked into the darkness. Fortunately, the first time I found the hole, I was moving slowly and was able to catch myself before I fell. But on my return trip I was running full steam ahead, so when I found the hole again, I was unable to catch myself. Bam! I fell flat and landed face down in the mud. Not knowing if the two guys were ready to pounce, I started to claw the wet ground in an effort to get away. Finally, I regained my footing and ran the short distance to the relative safety of the road where Suzy was waiting for me---laughing her head off.

It turns out she turned around to see what was taking me so long to return to safety and had seen the gleam of pure terror in my eyes as I clawed the earth in an effort to reach safety.

Fortunately for us, we reached the safety of our dorm and were able to calm down. We were sure, at the time that it was just fellow college students who were going to play a prank. We were just as equally sure that whoever it was would crack up laughing next time they saw me. If I saw someone fall flat on their face in front of me you wouldn't be able to keep me from laughing at them the next time I saw them.

Strangely enough, the laugh never came. And I still don't know who they were.

An easy ride

It was a gorgeous spring day, we wanted to be outside, and we decided that it was the perfect day for a bike ride. We did not want to push ourselves too hard, as it was one of our first rides of the year. So instead of opting for a mountain bike trail we headed out for a nice ride on the Chesapeake and Ohio Canal. The canal has a wonderful towpath that is flat, well maintained and is mostly shaded. It is the perfect place to go for an easy ride and it was our choice for that spring day. I put on shorts and a tee shirt and threw my hair into a ponytail. To top off my outfit, I put on a ball cap and threaded my ponytail through the hole in the back. I was ready to ride!

We quickly made our way to the canal and decided to head west on the 184-mile towpath. It did not take us long to get the bikes off the car. Within a few short minutes we headed off down the towpath toward the west. The birds were chirping and the weather was fantastic as we rolled along. It was one of those bike rides where we both felt as if our legs were made of pure muscle. We felt fantastic. We rode about 10 miles and then turned around to ride back to the car. We felt so amazing that we did not want to stop when we completed our out and back ride. We wanted to keep riding. No problem! We decided to ride about 4 miles eastwardly to the next access point. It would mean an extra 8 miles, but we were undaunted. Off we went!

It did not take us long to reach the next access point, which was a picnic area and boat ramp. Even though the fine weather had drawn a large amount of people utilizing the nearby picnic area, the boat ramp was empty. We decided to ride our bikes down to the boat ramp and check out the edge of the river before riding back to the car. That is when disaster struck!

The road to the boat ramp crosses over the canal and heads downhill to the water's edge. I did not pause when I got to the road but just veered off the canal onto that road and headed down the descent. I picked up speed, glorious speed! There is nothing like the feeling of a breeze washing over your body as you careen down a hill on your bike. I was picking up speed when the ball cap on my head flew off. It only took seconds for my ponytail to slip through the opening and the hat to fly off behind me in my wake. I jerked and my natural instinct was to look behind me for my now missing belonging. Maybe that was not the smartest thing to do on a bike, but that is exactly what I did. As I looked, I must have turned my handlebars and I could feel my bike waver out of control. I was in trouble and I knew it. Slow down my brain screamed at me. I grabbed the brakes and I pulled on them with all my might! That bike went from careening down the hill to a dead halt in a frighteningly short time.   Notice I said that the bike stopped. My body continued hurtling forward. Over the handlebars I went. Do not worry about me though. My face broke my fall.

Yes, I landed flat onto my face! I actually could see the arms on my glasses bend outward, for one split second before they fell to the ground beside me. (Yes, Oakley glasses really are that unbreakable.)   That is the only thing I remember from my time in the air and the actual crash.

I did not lose consciousness or anything like that, it all just happened so fast. I did not lay there for long and before Jason got to my side, I had already rolled to a sitting position. My face immediately started to hurt. All I could think about was my teeth. Please let my teeth be ok, I kept saying in my head. I believe that might be the first thing that I said to Jason. I remember trying to show him my teeth. Unfortunately, he could not see my teeth at first. I quite literally had a mouth full of dirt as my lip had curled outward and acted as a scoop to gather a mouth full of dirt. I began to spit in an effort to try to get the dirt out of my mouth. Jason handed me a bottle of water and told me to drink...but I had so much dirt that I kept rinsing my mouth out and spitting out black dirty water. Eventually he was able to see my teeth and somehow, miraculously; my teeth were fine. The rest of my face was not. Even as we sat there, my face began to swell. My right arm and leg had also obtained some wounds. I was a hot mess! I was also horribly embarrassed because there were people everywhere and I was sure that they had all seen my swan dive off my bike.

A stranger actually came over to see if I needed aid. By that time, Jason had retrieved tissues from my bag and I was dabbing at my injuries. We thanked the stranger but advised that we were ok. The stranger looked at me and said, "Just so you know, it was one spectacular fall"

Jason offered to let me sit at a picnic table and bring the car back to pick me up. However, I just wanted to get out of there! There were people everywhere and I was so embarrassed. So, as soon as I had wiped the dirt off of my face, dabbed up the blood from my leg and arm and steadied myself I got back on the bike. I actually rode out of there under my own steam. Seriously, there should have been a standing ovation for me as I rode away.

The 4 miles back to where we had parked the car were brutal for me. I was pretty banged up. As if every bone in my face hurting was not enough, I was also pretty messed up on the right side of my body. Blood was still dripping from those wounds. Those things were the least of my concerns though. During the ride back to the car, I started to feel some chest pain every time I took in a breath. I was petrified. I remember riding with silent tears pouring from my eyes. I was aware of Jason as he pedaled his bike as close to me as safety would allow. I could feel his concerned eyes on me. However, I did not say a word, not even when he would solicitously ask if I was ok. I would just nod my answer. I had one mission and that mission was to get back to the car.

Make it I did! We got back to the car and while I usually put my own bike on the roof rack, not that day. I was more than grateful to sit down in that car and let Jason take care of everything. I was so sore, but I was so proud of myself for pushing through and riding back.

Jason has since told me that it was one of the most terrifying moments of his life because he was sure that I had sustained serious injuries. Somehow, I managed to avoid serious injuries. For a few weeks, my face looked as if someone had beaten the heck out of me! Jason laughed and said he was almost embarrassed to go anywhere with me because people looked at him and assumed that he was someone that hit women.   My road rash and wounds healed relatively quickly. The inside of my mouth also suffered brush burn wounds as my lip must have curled back as I scrapped the pavement with my face. The chest pain? I did go to an urgent care for them to check out my ribs. There was no break; they said it was 'rib bruising'. I was told that the pain would eventually dissipate. They were right, it did; but it took months. I did not let my injuries stop me though. We were back on the bikes a week later (with plenty of Advil for me to dull the rib pain).

In answer to the question about helmets? We were utterly lax about wearing helmets at that point in our life. We would religiously wear a helmet when we were out on a mountain bike trail. However, on canal bike rides, we would relax that rule because it was a flat graded surface. What could go wrong? How badly could one get hurt on the canal? Let me tell you, you can get hurt pretty badly. I was lucky but I am well aware of how bad it could have been After this accident; we have made helmet use a mandatory rule!

Wear your helmet!!!

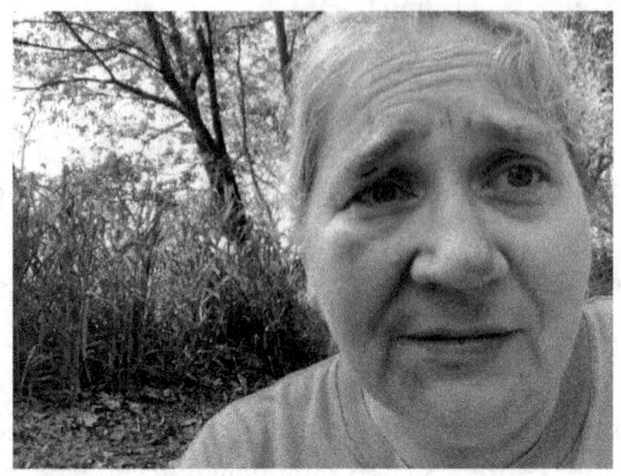

This was taken moments after I crashed. My face started to swell immediately!

Food

Weight loss revolves around food. We all know the saying that weight is lost in the kitchen and not the gym.   it only makes sense that I have encountered so many snafus and stories revolving around food.   Life is certainly interesting!

Hoss's cake

It was one of those days. I was tired and just didn't want to cook dinner. We decided to go to a local Steak House called Hoss's. If we went, I knew that I could order the salad bar and not only keep my eating in check but also stay within the confines of the caloric budget that I had set for my weight loss journey. Game on! We arrived and I was a champ! I was cognizant of everything that I put onto my plate. I counted every bite. I was doing great. I decided to head to the dessert area of the salad bar to get some sweet fruit for my dessert. I was that focused and I was doing great! But then I saw the Hoss Cake. It looked so delicious and it was cut in 1-inch square pieces. I knew what kind of hit my food budget would take if I indulged. I knew the points/calories for that piece of cake and I knew that I could afford to splurge! I carried that cake back to my table with awe and reverence. I slid into my booth and quickly picked up my fork. I hadn't had cake in quite some time and I was ready. My fork slide into the cake. Once the fork was loaded with cake I moved it into my mouth. Oh my word. It was heaven My eyes closed in ecstasy and I am sure a look of pure bliss was plastered on my face.   I swear, I could hear the angels singing the hallelujah chorus all around me! I savored each delicious bite of that one inch square of cake.   When I was done, I laid my fork down and the angels abruptly stopped singing. The bliss faded. I was left with the aftermath. I wanted the angels to sing again! I wanted the bliss back. I wanted it desperately. "Just one more piece," I said as I slid out of the booth. I brought back one more small square of cake and prepared for the glory that would be revealed to me as I ate the cake. But wait, the angels didn't sing when I ate the second piece. I wasn't filled with bliss. It wasn't heavenly! What was wrong! I wanted that! Quickly I went back for another piece of cake. Surely the next piece would bring back those feelings. Maybe the fourth piece? Fifth? I can't even tell you how many pieces of cake I ate that day as I tried to recapture the bliss and glory of those first few bites of something delicious.   It wasn't a day that I'm proud of. But it IS a day where I realized that I do have a food addiction. I was chasing the high. I was chasing the 'angels singing'. Time and time again over the years, I have chasing that bliss. When I find the blissful high, I have always incorrectly assumed that more and more of the same food will keep that bliss flowing over me. But in reality, the bliss and high comes from the first two or three bites. After that, the good feelings start to fade with each bite.

Pizza

In the height of losing weight (the first time) we would love to go to Pizza Hut. I would plan my pizza meals around my weight loss efforts. The meal after my weigh in at my Weight Watcher meeting was always my cheat meal. It gave me the freedom to have the foods and meals that were a bit higher in calories and/or points. It worked for me. For this reason, many nights I would leave my weight watchers meeting and pick up a pizza from Pizza Hut on the way home. I loved the thick crust pizza that they offer. That crust was delicious to me. I always eschewed the thin crust pizza. Who wants to eat pizza toppings on a crispy cracker? Not I!!!! But one day while I was tracking my food and looking at the nutritional facts for their pizza, I realized that I could save so many points/calories if I would switch to the thin crust pizza. It was such an efficient way to save in my food budget that I just had to make the switch. It never became my favorite and I always called it Cracker Crust Pizza and I would still occasionally splurge on the deep-dish crust.   But it was an amazing way to have my pizza and eat it too!

Empress Chicken

I had every intention of cooking and eating at home. EVERY intention. My intentions were so good that I had my food already noted in my daily tracker! I was going to have grilled chicken, roasted potatoes sprinkled with olive oil and rosemary, green beans, and fresh kiwi. It was all on paper and set it stone! I was set for success! What in the world happened when my husband got home and one of his first sentences was "Let's go to Chinese".   All of my plans went out the window. I quickly thought about what I had left in my food budget (I was counting points at that time). I actually knew I had the points to manage an order of Chicken and Broccoli. I was all set, so we decided to go! I got there, glanced at the menu and laid the menu aside. I knew what I was going to be ordering. It was all good. Well, my ex-husband was perusing the menu and must have felt weird about me just sitting there quietly. He suggested I actually look at the menu and try something new instead of staying with the same old same old.   I don't know why I didn't just say, "I know it's boring to you but I also know the points on my chicken and broccoli meal." NO, I didn't say that. I picked up the menu and found a dish that did sound REALLY good. The description actually sounded a lot like chicken and broccoli. Instead of broccoli, it was mixed veggies and water chestnuts though. It sounded yummy. So, I switched my plan and I was happy. I was happy until they sat the plate in front of me. When they sat the plate down in front of me, I just sat there and looked at it. To my credit after the waitress left our table, I did look at my ex-husband and say, "I can't eat this." What was the problem? It was deep fried chicken in a sauce mixed with the veggies. My ex was understanding. But it was ultimately my poor decision. I should have done a bit more investigative work before I ordered something new. I eventually smiled and said, "I'll just eat a small portion and we can take the rest home for your lunch tomorrow. I dished up a small portion for my dinner. The problem? Well, I tasted it and it was FABULOUS! It was so fabulous that I ate the portion on my plate. Oh my word it was so good and I wanted more. I dished up a some more and ate that too...and a little more... and then some more, until it was all gone. Heck, I practically licked that plate clean! (And found a new favorite dish.) I didn't do my research and just ordered without thought. I didn't win the weight loss journey battle that day.

A Rush

We were sitting at a restaurant and I was fairly confident that I would be able to navigate the experience without ruining the allotment of points/calories that I had for my meal. I had already decided upon ordering a vegetable platter and I knew that I could stay within my food budget with a vegetable platter. The waitress arrived at our table to greet us rather quickly. My dinner companion knew what to order and jumped in to place their lunch order while I was still opening the menu. Before I knew it, everyone was staring at me waiting for me to order! I felt rushed and put on the spot and my instincts took over. I had thought that I had built a strong set of habits over the time of my weight loss journey. But that day, when rushed and put on the spot I reverted back to the long buried and deeply ingrained habits.

I started to place my order. I ordered pickled beets as my first vegetable and a side salad with dressing on the side. Both were awesome and healthy choices. But then it all went downhill. "I'll take mashed potatoes with gravy." Definitely not the healthiest option, but not all was lost…. yet. However, don't breathe a sigh of relief just yet because my next words did me in. "Can I please have a side of Macaroni and Cheese." Still not convinced that I was too horrible with my ordering? When the waitress asked if I wanted a dinner roll, I said yes! That meal was a carbohydrate disaster! Oh boy, did it ever taste good going down though. I was rushed and didn't take the time I needed to calculate and plan. I ate my food, went home and THEN calculated my calories. What I found was shocking, demoralizing and upsetting.   I had messed up big time. There it was only shortly after lunchtime and I had already eaten most, if not all of my daily calories/points for the day. I had overeaten in terms of calories and in terms of carbohydrates. I didn't let my little snafu derail me. I planned a super healthy meal for dinner (all low-calorie vegetables) and I moved forward.

That day I learned a valuable lesson. Go into a restaurant with a strong plan. If you still need to fine tune that plan, do not allow yourself to be rushed. Take the time to calculate whatever you are counting, be it carbohydrates, calories, points, or fat (to name a few). Do not let those long buried habits have a chance to surface.

Chewing gum

Many people know that I love to bake. It is no secret that I enjoy it and happily volunteer to bake dessert for any function that I attend. I know that when I am in the kitchen baking something that my grin is as wide as a house. Baking is my happy place. But baking while on a weight loss journey? That is a different story! We had a few holiday functions to attend during one weekend so as normal, I volunteered (was volunteered) to bring cookie trays. With a sense of satisfaction, I planned an extravaganza day of cookie baking! NO problem! Oh wait, there was a problem, I was knee deep in my weight loss journey and didn't want to sidetrack my progress. I knew that I needed a plan! I decided early on that I would need to limit my taste testing. I decided that I would allow myself to have one bite of cookie dough and that I would allow myself to have one hot cookie fresh from the oven. Furthermore, I decided that while I was in the kitchen working that I would chew gum it would keep me from being tempted to pop a cookie into my mouth or snack during my long hours in the kitchen.

It worked fabulously, the chewing gum while baking was the best thing. When my gum got stale, I swapped it out for a new piece. When the time came for my two planned indulgences (one bite of cookie dough and one fresh cookie), I took the gum out of my mouth and enjoyed my indulgence before promptly replacing the piece of gum. It was wonderful. I was cognizant of something already in my mouth, and it eliminated so much of my snacking and taste testing. But that day made me realize exactly how much mindless nibbling really occurs whilst in the kitchen. Time and time again I found myself popping in a little piece of this or a little bite of that. Immediately, the essence of the cookie would interact with the flavor of the gum in my mouth creating an odd taste in my mouth. That odd taste is what constantly pulled me back to reality and made me realize that without even knowing it, I had put something in my mouth to eat. I learned that day that baking is a landmine for me because I don't even realize how much mindless nibbling I do!

Save more eat more

There must have been something in the air to make me forget myself. We stopped at Waffle House for breakfast one morning while we were out. I knew what I was going to get. I was going to get one waffle. I knew exactly how it would affect my food budget and I had planned accordingly! No problem! We sat down and the first thing I saw was the sign that said, "We now have chocolate chip waffles". Oh my, that sounded like heaven here on earth! I debated. I really did, I debated long and hard. However, I finally decided to go ahead, take the hit on my daily food budget and live on the edge. I was getting a chocolate chip waffle! Satisfied with my decision, I sat back to wait for the server. With nothing else to do, I looked down at the menu. I was stunned. Did you know that you paid 2.35 for one waffle and only paid 99 cents for a second waffle (prices were at the time that this occurred, I am sure that it is quite a bit more now). 99 cents for double the food. The server came right after I saw this incredible deal. Before I knew it, I had ordered a double chocolate chip waffle. Before you think that double means just a little bit more, NO, it is two whole waffles instead of one. I could have put one in a to-go box and taken it home. For 99 cents, I could have left one uneaten. I could have done those things. However, I did not. I ate every darn bit of both of those waffles. I enjoyed every bite too!

I may think I have control of my food choices, but this story just goes to show me that when push comes to shove that I still fail. I honestly do not know what happened to me that day. I saw the great deal and before I could really think over my actions and the consequences, I blurted out that I wanted it. I really did not want it and I definitely did not need it. The best I can guess is that I was overwhelmed with the incredible deal and the untimely fast arrival of the server. I would like to hope that had I had a few more minutes that I would have come to my senses before ordering the double waffle to 'save money'. These restaurants come up with incredible deals. Pay 99 cents more and get double the food. It is only a great deal if you need that extra food. For the average person it is a waste of money because we do not really need that extra food.

The steakhouse Runs

"Why don't we eat out?" were the words out of my partner's mouth. I moaned internally. It was not that I did not want to go out to eat. I mean, who wouldn't want to step out the kitchen and let someone else do the cooking and the clean up! I am also a bit of a push over, so I gave my approval and off we went. My internal angst came from the fact that we were going to be going to a buffet style restaurant. In the previous weeks, I had been doing amazing with my efforts to lose weight. I did not want an innocent sounding 'eat out' event to derail me. You see, a buffet can very quickly be the kiss of death to any semblance of eating healthy. There is all manner of delicious food on a buffet; foods that will sideline any weight loss plan. I was determined though. I was NOT going to let this buffet style restaurant win. Luckily, we had frequented this restaurant in the past so I had an idea what would be involved. I thought for a few minutes and came up with my plan. I would say no to the delicious yeast rolls. I would turn my back on the mammoth dessert bar. I would not even look at the vats of macaroni and cheese and I would turn up my nose at anything fried! I could do this! I gathered every ounce of my willpower and determination as we headed into that restaurant.

Let me tell you, I was a brick wall when it came to anything unhealthy. I held firm. I only ate what I had planned to eat. I filled my plate with all manner of vegetables. I was on top of the world. I was so proud of myself. I sat at that table feeling the most incredible sense of pride at my success. Vegetables had never tasted so good! I managed to avoid the decadent looking desserts. Instead, I opted for fresh fruit. I was a girl on fire with my decisions and I knew it!

After dinner, we decided to walk through the mall. Victorious over my raging success with my food choices I was super excited to add some steps and miles to my legs for a bit more activity. I was totally on board with making my evening out a success on every aspect of healthy living.

The disaster struck about half way into our walk through the mall. My stomach started to grumble a bit. Then it started to roll and churn. Finally, my stomach decided to give it up and it went into full out spasms and contractions of pain. I cannot even begin to tell you how fast this hit me! I could literally feel the beads of sweat on my forehead. I looked at my dinner companion and through clenched teeth, I said, "I need the bathroom and I need it now."   There was no hesitation on his part. I think the lack of hesitation was due to the sickly green pallor that had tinged my complexion.   I was sick and he knew it. We hustled off toward the bathrooms, which were of course at the other end of the mall. The whole time I was praying to make it. At that point, I honestly did not know at which end of my body the explosion would occur. I just knew I had to get to the bathroom.

I made it. I was never so happy to plop my behind on a public toilet seat. I feel sorry for anyone in the bathroom at the time of my explosion. I was in there for a while until my body had dispelled every ounce of badness in my body. When I left the bathroom, I had no trace of stomach problems. I was a-ok, just nervous that it would come back!

What in the world had caused my explosive illness though? It was not until a few weeks later when we went back to that same restaurant that I realized what had happened. On that fateful evening, I had made incredible choices by eating all sorts of vegetables. I had filled my plate to the brim with 'healthy choices". What I had not taken into consideration was all of the butter and fats that had been used in the preparation of those 'healthy' vegetables. Those vegetables were literally floating in a sea of butter/margarine in the steam trays at that buffet. While eating at home I utilize healthy methods of cooking vegetables.   In other words, my vegetables are not swimming in fat at home. My body was not used to the quantity of butters and fats and it rebelled.   Lesson learned!

Where's the Bread

I was super determined to be successful, even though we were planning on eating dinner out a restaurant. I had patronized the locally owned steakhouse previously so I knew the pitfalls of eating healthy at this establishment.   My plan was to order a salad and water. I was perfectly fine with that option. (Not ordering an entrée was actually common for me as at that time I was mostly eating vegetarian).   My first possible pitfall was in the fact that I knew from previous experiences that they did not have many healthy options for a salad dressing. They had absolutely none other than a simple oil and vinegar, which to be perfectly honest; I do not like. Therefore, that was a huge potential pitfall. The second pitfall would be the delicious bread the table that they always brought to the table. That one was going to be quite difficult. I knew that the warm bread would be steaming and casting its amazing aroma across our table. For a self-proclaimed carb-o-holic, that could mean disaster! Regardless of those two huge potential pitfalls, I was determined to be successful. Therefore, I created a more detailed plan!

The first thing I did was to run into the grocery store that was adjacent to the steakhouse while my dinner companion went in to get us a table. I knew what I was looking for and it was only moments after we were assigned our table that I joined the party at our table. What did I buy at the grocery store?   I bought a bottle of salad dressing. I knew that my healthy options would be next to none at the steakhouse, so I took in my own.   Yes, I placed my purchased bottle of a healthier salad dressing on the table beside my silverware. Was there embarrassment at carrying in my own salad dressing? Not even a smidgen! There was a huge sense of pride though. I had made a healthy decision for myself and I was proud! With my healthier choice for a salad dressing, I had set myself up for success.

The bread was a much more complex issue. The easiest option would be to tell the wait staff that we do not want any bread. If it is not on the table the problem is totally fixed! The issue comes into play when you are dining with other people. Those people may want bread and it is not fair to impose my limitations on other. When that is the case, it really does rely on good old-fashioned will power to avoid the bread! Luckily was with me that night. My dinner companion was perfectly fine with refusing the bread.

Since I already had a plan for my meal, it did not long to order our food. The wait staff walked away and we commenced with the companionship of sharing a meal. We were quite a few minutes into our conversation before I remembered that we had agreed to tell the waiter that we did not want bread.   We discussed this overlook and agreed that we would simply tell any wait staff that arrived at our table with bread to take it away. Problem solved!

Our food came out relatively quickly and we smiled as we looked at the food before us. I looked up and saw that the waiter had deposited the food on the table but had not brought any bread. Even better, right? Problem solved, almost like divine intervention! I honestly have no clue what happened to me. I must have been temporarily insane because when the waiter asked, "Do you need anything else?" I quickly said, "You forgot our bread!"

As soon as the words were out of my mouth, I knew that I had committed a major mistake. My eyes got big as saucers and I was rendered speechless.   I looked across the table at my dinner companion. Their mouth was literally resting on their chest as their face formed a complete mask of shock! We were both in such a stupor at my comment that we did not have a chance to stop the waiter before they turned and walked away. Because of course, they had gone to get the forgotten bread. When the waiter returned, they were so apologetic for forgetting our breadbasket. I could only smile as they happily announced that they had given us double the amount since they had forgotten.

What in the world happened to me? I do not know. I opened my mouth and those words just came out! I would like to say that I was able to avoid that double dose of warm steamy bread. However, I cannot make that claim. At least I held firm and used my purchased salad dressing!

Counting Chips

I had just enough room in my food budget to have a snack! I knew what we had in the kitchen available to snack on. I was so tickled to be able to have some potato chips. Specifically, we had Pringles potato chips. I was so excited and could not wait to sink my teeth into my snack. It was so tempting to rip open the can and dive in headfirst! However, I knew that I had just enough room in my food budget for one serving of these coveted chips. I had to eat my snack wisely. Carrying the whole can of Pringles Potato Chips into the living room would NOT be wise. I knew that I would open the can and eat my serving but then continue with 'just one more' until surprisingly, the whole can would be gone. That was not going to happen to me. I was a girl on a mission and I was going to eat my serving and nothing else. I was not going to ruin my upcoming weigh in. I stood in the dimly lit kitchen and counted out those potato chips. I handled them reverently and carefully. I was savoring every moment of the experience. Once my serving size count was complete, I closed the lid to the Pringles can and I picked up my stack of potato chips. It was time to enjoy. Let me tell you, I was so proud of myself for my strength and determination with this snack.

I moved into the living room and settled onto the couch to partake of my 'legal' snack while watching the television. Pringles stack so nicely, so I had just carried my stack into the living room with me. I carefully balanced my stack of potato chips onto my thigh and began to eat. They tasted so good! I was not paying attention to how many I had eaten. After all, I had counted them before I began so I did not have to worry. I knew that I could just eat until they were gone. That is when disaster struck!

I have loved each and every cat that I have been blessed to have in my life. I really have! However, that night, I did not love my cat. You see, she jumped up onto the couch and onto my lap. She landed directly onto my stack of Pringles. Oh yes, it was a direct hit and those glorious potato chips could not withstand the tidal force of my cat. The remaining chips shattered into a million pieces.

I looked down in disbelief and I started to cry. Oh yes, I did cry over some crushed and newly unrecognizable potato chips. Sure, I could have gone into the kitchen and grabbed some undamaged potato chips to replace my ruined ones. However, how many would I need in order to replace what had been damaged without ruining my food budget? Had I eaten four potato chips? Maybe I had eaten ten potato chips. Should I possibly short change myself and only get one or two potato chips or should I go big, get a handful, and thereby possibly ruin my perfect day of eating? I should be ashamed to admit that the crushed Pringles brought me to tears. I ended up choosing to error on the side of caution that night. I did not get any more potato chips to replace what the flying cat had damaged. I was feeling super strong and determined that night. I liked that feeling of pride in myself and I did not want to give that up, even though I brought me to tears.

It's not in what you eat

I was sitting at my weight watchers meeting. As with every meeting (at that time at least) the leader started by opening the floor for everyone to share their weight losses for the week, the victories of the week and even the failures. I was one of the first people to volunteer to share. I had lost 2.4 pounds for the week. My total loss for Weight Watchers was 50.8 pounds and my total loss overall was 110 pounds. I was super tickled and proud of myself.

The next person to speak was a gentleman who decided to share about how he had a non-scale victory because he had gone to a buffet and instead of the cheesy carbohydrate laden foods, he chose Brussel sprouts.   Great job!   That is a great non-scale victory indeed.   One of the women in the group turned up her nose and made the comment. "That is huge because I cannot stand Brussel Sprouts." I couldn't help but laugh in agreement.

The weight watcher leader used the Brussel sprouts to segue into a conversation to remind us about the zero-point foods that were currently on the list (at that time there was not a whole bunch). The Brussel sprout hater asked what to do if she did not like those foods though.   I started to laugh even more. You see, I liked very few of the zero-point foods.   I was ok with sauerkraut and green beans. Sometimes I was able to choke down raw carrots and broccoli. Salads were ok, but only if they had lots of salad dressing and cheese, which pretty much negates the zero-point aspect.   I made no secret of my distaste for those zero points foods during that meeting.

 The newer people in the room were all sitting there with their jaws dropped; because we had literally just celebrated my 50/110 pound weight loss, (I had a good leader that celebrated both my WW number and my total number even though I only got rewards for my WW number). I looked at them and said, "I am a testament to the fact that you don't have to eat only healthy foods. You just have to make better choices and eat less when you make that choice to eat something that is less healthy. That is really what it's all about. I KNOW I could eat a donut...but then I would use up all my points and I would not be able to eat the rest of the day. That is not a good choice for me. Nor is it a healthy one."

 One girl was like "Well what about pizza?"

I started to laugh and I answered honestly. "I eat pizza. Not a version of pizza that is a healthy version. I eat real restaurant purchased pizza. I just do not do it every other day. I do not even do it once a week. But when I do have pizza, I manage what I eat the rest of the day to accommodate that indulgence." I looked at the woman that had asked about pizza and I said, "If you look at my food tracker, you will see that I had Pizza two weeks ago and at my next weigh in I still lost 1.5 pounds."

The room was buzzing with this revelation. One person jumped in and said, "For me it's not pizza, its Chinese food".

All I could do was laugh as I show them my food tracker. You see, the day after we had pizza, we ate out at a Chinese restaurant and that was the week where I lost 1.5 pounds. If you want something, you will make the accommodations and adjustments to make it work.

The Fickle Friend

As an adult, I am the person that has been primarily responsible for the cooking and clean up. You can say that the kitchen is 100% my domain. I enjoy cooking and baking so I do not mind the aspect of creating food at all. The cleanup part though could go away. However, it is part of the process so I take care of it. Sometimes being in the kitchen is difficult when it comes to eating healthy and properly. I have to guard against nibbling on food when I am cooking and baking. I have to watch out for all of those bites licks and tastes that we take in the kitchen because they add up! I had been doing really well with the impulse to nibble and taste whilst in the kitchen until the self-control is thrown out the window.

Dinner was over and I was alone in the kitchen cleaning up. There were leftovers from dinner but I did not want to keep them. What we had eaten was something that I knew would not hold over well as a leftover. Therefore, I planned to throw the leftovers away. I grabbed the bowl of leftover food and walked to the garbage can. With one hand, I started to tilt the bowl over the trash can. I had a serving spoon in my other hand to aid in the removal of the food into the garbage. The smell of my delicious dinner wafted up to greet my nose and my hand paused before even a drop of food had left the bowl. "I better get one more bite," I told myself. I used the spoon to scoop out a bite. Oh, my word it tasted so good. "Just one more," the voice in my head said. That is how I found myself to be standing over the garbage can, greedily shoveling food into my mouth. I did not need that food. There was no way that I was hungry. I did not have the room in my food budget for the food. Yet, I continued to eat even while I was poised over the garbage ready to dump the food. Eventually I did gather my willpower and I dumped the contents of that bowl. But not before I ate what amounted to a complete extra serving of that food.

I knew what I was doing. The entire time that I was standing over the garbage spooning food into my mouth, I was berating myself. I lost all aspects of myself control there for a little bit. Self-control is a fickle friend and that day it disappeared for a bit.

But it's Zero

I was a new member at Weight Watchers and I was determined to get it right. I poured over the books and pamphlets. I scoured cookbooks. I spent hours looking at different foods. I wanted to get this weight off and get it off for the last time! I played with the numbers. I was playing by the rules. If I ate a cup of something and it said it was 6 points, I counted it as six points.

At this point in Weight Watchers history, they did not have the extensive zero points food lists that they have now. However, we all knew about certain foods that were so low in calories and fat and everything else that goes into making a weight watchers point that they ended up to be zero calories for one serving of said item. There were a few out there. We could eat celery! Yes, celery was of course a freebie! However, I am not a big fan of celery. Sure, chopped and cooked in something it is fine. However, raw on its own is a definite no go for me. For me that is yucky! I did not like many of those so-called free foods and I honestly refused to eat something if I did not like it!

Luckily, I found a few foods that actually came out to be zero points! Ok, I found two things, to be exact. Not matter that it was only two things, I was absolutely ecstatic! I started to throw those two foods in my lunch. What were they? Sauerkraut and green beans! Yummy right? But hey, they were foods that I actually did like! I packed those two things in my lunchbox every darn day of the week. Every. Darn. Day. I did that for about a year (or more)!

It was an amazing year. That year of eating sauerkraut and green beans was the year that I lost a significant amount of weight during my first round of losing 100 plus pounds. I know that filling up on those free foods (low calories) versus eating higher point/calorie foods was instrumental to my success! But seriously, every day?

I made it through that period intact and I did not go crazy from the lack of variety. I did end up with a different side effect. For years afterward I could not stand the smell or taste of those two foods! It was probably at least 10 years before I started to willingly eat those zero points foods again and even to this day, I don't mind them but they are no longer favorite options for me. But hey, the sauerkraut and green beans served their purpose at the time!

Sauerkraut Bomb

I had been eating a lot of sauerkraut. It was such a low-calorie food that I could use that to fill up without breaking the food budget bank. It sounds crazy, but it was working for me and I was not too ashamed to tell people my secret. I mentioned it in passing quite a few times. I didn't mention the fact that I was not eating big vats of it in one sitting. I also didn't mention that; as my grandmother used to say, "Sauerkraut will clean you out". (You get the drift, I'm sure!)

It was Zumba night and I was so excited. I loved Zumba nights! I went to Zumba a few times a week and had made some great friends in the class. Most nights were normal dance Zumba but one night a week, we were doing Sentao, which was a dance choreography that used a chair. (Do not let the chair thing fool you. This class was HARDER than any other was!) We always jockeyed for spots on the dance floor close to each other so that we could encourage each other. We would always say a few words to each other between songs or at any breaks in the class. This night was no different. I was positioned beside my one friend and we began our workout. It was midway through the workout and there was a short break. I looked over at my friend. She dropped to her chair. She reclined against the back of the chair, almost dramatically so. She looked over and me. I could see a look of unease in her eyes. I did not know what it was about until she said "I followed your lead and I had a big can of sauerkraut for dinner before class." She clutched her stomach as he continued, "My stomach is just rolling".

I started to laugh and just had to ask her how much she ate. "I was really hungry so I got the biggest container they had". She went on with the workout. I do not know how! However, between songs she let me know that the sauerkraut had done its job before she came to the class and she had 'cleaned out her insides" and she thought she was good. But, as soon as she started to move in the class, she could feel her stomach clenching and she knew that she had to go to the bathroom again.   She left the class two or three times to run to the bathroom. Somehow, she made it through the workout!

A workout was not all she got that day. She also learned that there are certain foods you want to limit. It may sound like a great deal, but a little will go a long way!

It tastes like Dirt

I packed my lunch for work. I smiled to myself as I put my healthy choices into my lunch box. I had packed the same things in my lunches for the previous weeks. More importantly, I had been doing fantastic with my weight loss. I was on a roll and I was proud of myself for the food choices that I made when I packed my lunch. It was quite nutritious. There were some raw carrots and I had some yogurt. It was a healthy and nutritious lunch!

The problem came when I started to eat it. I started with the yogurt because yogurt was not my thing. I knew that I did not like yogurt when I bought it and I knew I did not like yogurt when I packed it in my lunch for the day! However, all of the healthy living and weight loss gurus expounded on how yogurt was 'the thing' to eat if you were trying to lose weight. So there I was with yogurt for lunch, all for the sake of being healthy. I plunked my spoon into the container of yogurt and I ate that yogurt. Before you ask, I did try different brands and I did buy different flavors to try to make it more palatable. However, to my palate, there isn't much about yogurt worth eating! Yet there I was eating it, spoonful after spoonful! I nearly gagged with each bite!   I was so happy when that yogurt was done! It was time to move on to the next item in my lunchbox.

 Ahh the carrots. I opened my bag of raw carrots and took a bite. I could hear the crunch reverberate through my head. I slowly started to chew. And I chewed some more. Wow, raw carrots take a long time to chew! It gave me a lot of time to think and I had an epiphany right there as I ate my lunch. I sat there thinking about how I really do not like raw carrots. I had known for years that I don't really like to eat raw carrots frequently. I personally feel as if they taste like dirt (Yes, I have the palate of a toddler)! The Epiphany was in the fact that here I was eating a lunch that I absolutely abhorred, all in the name of being healthy because someone had told me that these items were the end all be all weight loss foods. Why was I doing that to myself?   Eating food you hate is not living life. It is not sustainable for a lifelong quest to be healthy. During that lunch break I realized that if I want to make this new lifestyle a permanent change that I needed to stop forcing myself to eat foods that did not appeal to me at all.

I did not even finish that lunch I chucked those carrots right in the garbage and decided that I would rather go hungry than eat another bite! I cannot even begin to tell you how much joy was in my soul when I threw those carrots in the garbage can. I do occasionally eat a raw carrot or some yogurt, but I refuse to make it a staple in my life. But hey, maybe someday I will grow to really like them! So never say never!

Red Meat

I was on a roll with my healthy eating! Bad food was not passing my lips. Fast food was a thing of the past. I rarely ate meat and when I did, it was chicken or turkey. I was doing fabulous and my body was loving it! I was never tempted with stopping at the multitude of fast-food restaurants that I passed on a daily basis. I didn't miss it and I didn't want it.

I was out and about running errands one fateful day. I was not at all tempted to stop for food. However, I was in desperate need to use the bathroom.   What better place than a fast-food restaurant? I swung into the first place I saw, a Wendy's. The aroma of hamburger and bacon grease hit me when I walked through the door. Something happened to me when I smelled it. For the first time in ages, my mouth salivated at the thought of eating red meat. Fast food at that!   I hightailed it directly to the bathroom and took care of my business. My mind was whirling around in circles. I hadn't had red meat in at least a year or two, but the smell of the burgers had blown me away and I could think of nothing other than actually sinking my teeth into a burger. Maybe it was memories of all the times that my family had gone to Wendy's whilst growing up. Maybe I was just hungry and I had not realized it. Whatever it was, I couldn't get the prospect of having a hamburger out of my mind.

There was no reason why I couldn't get a cheeseburger. My reasons for not eating meat were not based on any health plan or diet. I had simply stopped eating meat for personal and humanitarian reasons a few years earlier. I washed my hands and walked out of the bathroom. In my mind I was still dithering back and forth. I didn't really need a cheeseburger. I had eaten lunch and it was nowhere near time for dinner yet. I just really wanted to taste a cheeseburger.

I caved. Instead of heading out the door to the car, I caved. I headed to the counter and ordered. Out of respect to my healthy lifestyle and my weight loss efforts, I did only order a Junior Cheeseburger instead of a multi-patty full sized version. I took that first bite and it wasn't bad. It tasted so odd after all those years of eschewing red meat. I took another bite and then a third bite.

Three bites is all it took. My stomach began to flip from the unaccustomed food and grease. It lay in my stomach like a 10-pound weight.   I threw the rest of the burger away and walked out of the restaurant. I'm sure that there was nothing wrong with the cheeseburger. My body was just not used to that kind of food.

I felt queasy for the next few hours but it finally passed. That was the last time I ordered a cheeseburger for a long time. I had no qualms about remaining red meat free at that time.

Fast Food

I was on a healthy kick and going strong. My food intake was healthy. I was not eating very much unhealthy foods and my body was loving how it felt. Everything was going well until stress hit and then it all went belly up and boy was it painful!

My mom had suffered a stroke and my emotions were all over the place in the first weeks and months following the stroke. The first week in particular was difficult as she had been airlifted to a hospital that specialized in strokes and neurological issues. This hospital was 4 hours away.   I had been eating so healthy but the stress beat me down. In hindsight, I should have packed some snacks for the hotel and for healthy options to eat in my car while traveling. But that was the last thing that I was thinking about.   It was inevitable that I end up eating at a fast-food restaurant while traversing the turnpike.

The food tasted great! It was the after effects that got me. I was totally not used to eating fast food. Fast food is greasy goodness. Fast food is lower quality food than I was used to eating. Fast food did not sit well in my belly! My stomach began to gurgle. My stomach began to cramp. I squeezed my sphincter muscles together and I started to pray that the miles would pass quickly to the next travel plaza on that turnpike.   I made it, but it sure did a number on me!

One would think that I had learned my lesson, but that very night I struggled again. I had gotten to the hospital and hightailed it directly to the ER where mom was being seen. Her helicopter ride had been much faster than my drive, so they had already reevaluated her and we were waiting for a room to be open as she was being admitted. I settled in to wait with her. We waited and waited and waited. The evening passed and it was well after midnight. Mom could see that I was ready to drop and insisted that I head to the nearby hotel. I made sure the hospital had my information and drove the few blocks to the hotel where reservations had been made in my name. I hadn't eaten since that fateful fast food in the early afternoon and I was hungry. What do you eat at 1 in the morning? Vending machine food and the snacks in the hotel shop it was. Junk food! Another meal that lay heavy in my stomach! I would have been better going to bed hungry. Instead, I went to bed sick!

Big Brown Eyes

I was driving down the interstate minding my own business. I was on a day trip to see some sights with a friend and we were ready to have some fun. But first we had to get to our destination. I wasn't speeding, just going a nice steady speed in the slow lane. We were talking about mundane things and singing along with the music that played from the radio. I noticed a large truck pulling up on my left to pass me. I didn't think anything of it. That's what happens on the interstate. The front of the truck passed and the trailer pulled alongside me. I turned my head to the left and that is when I saw that the truck was full of cows. Cows that were most likely on their way to the slaughter house. They were all riding in that truck and looking out at freedom. I could see their gentle brown eyes looking at me and their eyes held a look of sadness that shook me to the core. Those cows knew that they were going nowhere good and my heart broke. (Yes, it was heartbroken for a cow!)

I held eye contact with those gentle eyes until the truck moved too far away. There was no thought, no hesitation and no question. I turned to my friend and said, "I can't eat beef anymore."

And just like that I dropped beef from my daily diet. For the most part it was an easy decision that I had no problem upholding. During the first year or two I would occasionally crave a cheeseburger. But the cravings were usually fast and fleeting and sparked by seeing a restaurant that I knew served good burgers. I didn't eat red meat for years!

My family was not overly surprised at my declaration and not just because of my feelings for the gentle eyed cows. Growing up, I had gone through quite a few years where I ate limited meat. I well remember many nights where my parents and brother were eating from plates laden with meat while I sat with jars of peanut butter and jelly beside my plate. I would still eat the side dishes but had no desire for the meat. It honestly wasn't until college that I started to eat meat more regularly. I ate meat regularly for about 15 years, until I was in my early to mid-30's and I saw that gentle eyed cow in the truck on the way to slaughter.

About a year or two after I gave up beef it struck again. I was reading an article about pigs. The article discussed how pigs are actually a rather smart animal that literally go insane in the conditions that many are being raised in. They go so crazy that they bite off their own tails. I wasn't sure (and still am not) of the validity of that claim, but it was enough for me. Pork had to go! Pork was a bit difficult for me. I do like bacon and I do like pepperoni. For that reason, I never really fully gave up pork. I would try to substitute turkey versions of those foods when possible. I would nix bacon on sandwiches when I went out. I would try to avoid pepperoni.   But occasionally I would cave and eat it, usually I would say, "I'm not really convinced that pepperoni/bacon is meat" I had waitresses, family members and friends give me odd looks when I made that declaration!   I had to occasionally stop and say, "It's a joke! I know where pepperoni and bacon came from!"

I was happy with my lifestyle that didn't include pork or beef. I did not miss it at all. I had never liked seafood so that left me with chicken and turkey as the sole meat products in my diet. It was working for me. Most days I would not eat any meat at all and only had chicken or turkey once or twice a week.   I was feeling amazing.

It was a few years after I had pretty much stopped eating pork that I met up with friends at a restaurant in Lancaster County, PA. It as a buffet style restaurant and I was ok with that as I knew that they had lots of meatless options that I could pick from.   I was filling my plate when I saw the piles of sliced ham. It smelled so delicious. It looked stupendously good. I held out my plate and watched with a smile as the piece of ham slide onto it. I was grinning as I sat down at the table. The ham was admittedly the first thing that I put into my mouth.   It was all I could do to keep from spitting it out.   Oh my word, it was horrid! I didn't say a word as everyone else at the table chewed their pieces of ham and raved about how delicious it was! That is when I realized that I had developed a completely different palate. Meat no longer was appealing to my taste buds! I pushed the meat aside and went back to my meatless options.

I happily went on with my relatively meatless life. I had no reason to go back to eating meat. Furthermore, as the years passed, I realized that the less I ate meat, the more I abhorred it.

In 2014 I ended up moving in with my parents as I went through a divorce. I was on the go a lot and ended up eating a lot of my dinners out as I was heading to and from exercise classes and evenings out with friends. Every once in a while, I would have an evening home with my parents and I would get to enjoy a dinner with them. I could only laugh at the meals I ate that my mom prepared.   On one of my first nights home my mom was so excited to have me there and she made tacos! Lots of hamburger taco meat was there for me to fix my taco!   I ended up eating a shell with cheese and some toppings and just laughed about it as I knew that she had forgotten my eating habits.

Mom started to get better and a while later I was once again home for dinner. Mom was so proud of herself as she served up dinner. She had made spaghetti and meatballs. She was so excited to tell me all about how she had made the meatballs, they were in a different bowl, and I would not have to be confronted with them mixed in my sauce. (That is love, isn't it?)   I dished up my portion for dinner and sat at the table ready to dig in. I took one bite and I stopped. It tasted quite foul! I looked around but everyone else was loving it. Immediately I knew what the problem was. Mom had cooked the meatballs in the pan and removed them to the bowl for everyone else. She had then used the same pan to make the spaghetti sauce. The same pan that she didn't wash. The pan that was coated with the juices and grease from the meatballs. Ohhh yeah, it tainted that sauce something fierce! But mom was trying! I knew she would get it eventually.

Before mom 'got it' though, I meat Jason and we started to date. I managed to keep up my meatless existence with him. He certainly didn't care what I ordered or what I ate. However, he made a comment. "Stick with me and you will be eating meat in 6 months." I laughed because how was he going to get me to eat meat. At that point it had been close to 10 years since I had eaten meat on a regular basis.

I don't know how he did it. He never said a word. He never encouraged me to eat something. It was never discussed. But within 6 months, I was eating meat every day!

The pumpkin Diet

I was working with a gal that was great fun! She was always trying something different, trying something new or coming up with some outlandish comment. She made the workday go by so fast. It was never a dull moment and I never laughed at work quite as much as I did when I worked with Leslie.

It was a spring day when Leslie decided that she needed to lose weight. Of course, she didn't say it quite that way. I am sure it was worded in a more interesting and unique way.   Leslie dove into this weight loss mission with her usual offbeat manner. She was full of plans and fun. She was going to lose this weight and she was going to lose it her way! I was honestly tickled about her personal mission for two reasons. The first reason is that it would give me an extra accountability partner! I knew that surrounding myself with like-minded people was instrumental to my own success. The second reason was purely for my own entertainment. I knew that with whatever she did, that it would be a complete hoot.

Leslie did not disappoint me on the entertainment value. However, I was a bit shocked at how quickly it came about.   It was a Friday when she made her bold declaration about being healthy and losing weight. We went home for the weekend and when she came back, she had a story to tell!

It was a Saturday afternoon and she was deep into reading a book. She was getting hungry. She headed to the kitchen, with no real plan of action in terms of what to eat. She was actually a bit annoyed to have to set her book down. She wanted something quick and easy so that she could get back to her book. But she was also trying to eat in a way that would cause her to lose weight. She didn't know what to do.   She stepped into the pantry to see what was available. She was looking for quick and easy first but she was also looking at nutritional labels to find something that was lower in calories. She finally settled on a can of vegetables. She could pop the can open, quickly reheat the food and it would be relatively healthy. She was determined! Her weight loss journey had just started. She wanted weight loss and she wanted it now! She decided to peruse the labels on all the vegetables and simply eat the vegetable with the lowest caloric value. She was busy going through the labels when her eyes fell upon the can of pumpkin puree. She checked the nutritional label and this was the lowest calories of all the foods.   She admitted to being a bit worried since she had never eaten raw pumpkin puree before. However; In her words, "I like pumpkin pie, so I figured pumpkin puree should taste pretty good"

Her choice was made. Pumpkin Puree it was. She opened the can and sat down with a spoon and her book to enjoy her lunch. The first bite wasn't that bad, not good but edible. But with each bite, she could feel it settle in her stomach. She only made it about 3-4 spoons full of the puree before her stomach was completely done with food.   "Pumpkin puree is not at all like pumpkin pie," she boldly declared on Monday at work.   The taste and feel of the puree were enough to drive her out of the kitchen. It took all desire to eat away from her. Her stomach was still feeling the effects of that pumpkin puree hours later.

As horrible as the experience sounded, Leslie was tickled with what had happened "I didn't eat anything the rest of the day," She happily announced. "I have decided that anytime I am hungry I will just go eat a few spoons full of pumpkin puree and it will make me not eat the rest of the day!"   Yes, she had discovered her new weight loss plan!   Did it work?   Who knows, her diet days only lasted a few more days before she was onto her next crusade!

Downfall Wedding

I had just reached my goal weight! I was super excited! I felt amazing. I looked amazing and I was feeling on top of the world. I was excited to buy a new dress and travel to Indiana for my friend's wedding. I was combining the wedding with a visit to my brother and his family as he also lived in Indiana at that time. I knew that a vacation would pose some obstacles in terms of my weight loss /maintenance efforts. I was not worried. I had a plan. I was going to stick with my eating plan and exercise religiously! I took exercise equipment with me. At that time Dance Dance Revolution was a bit thing on the Xbox and I took my floor mats. I took my aerobic steps and step aerobics videos. I took my running shoes. I took it all! We were going to be gone for 10 days and I was going to come home victorious!

The wedding was the first stop on our trip to the Midwest. I was feeling confident and ready to conquer this vacation. I was wearing a size 8 dress. Size eight! Nothing was going to keep me from wearing that dress over and over again! The wedding was absolutely gorgeous and I was so honored to be able to attend this wedding.   We traversed to the wedding reception and we settled in to have a good time. I was so strong. I chose my food carefully. I wasn't going to let a buffet of food derail me! I was doing amazing!   But then it was time for the cake! Cake is a downfall of mine! I enjoy cake and I REALLY love cake with a lot of icing. It's no secret that if given a choice, I will go for a piece with the most icing!   I actually was ready to resist this wedding cake!   But then the bride sauntered by our table. She had also been on a weight loss journey (one of my main accountability partners actually) and had also reached her goal weight. After greeting me and hearing that I was refraining from eating any wedding cake she said one thing to me, "It's my wedding...you have to have wedding cake!"   Now who am I to argue! Plus, there is folklore out there that says eating wedding cake brings good luck to everyone! I needed luck!   So off I went to the cake table to get myself a piece of wedding cake.   I am proud to say that I just had that one piece of cake....that day.

I was so good with my choices at that wedding. I had only that one piece of cake, and honestly, it was a small piece! There shouldn't have been a problem. Except that there was a huge problem. I had just managed to reach my lifetime goal with weight watchers a few weeks earlier. I had been doing amazing with my weight loss. One of the keys to my success had been to recognize the fact that I have a food addiction and I had chosen to simply avoid the foods that most triggered my addiction. One of the foods that trigged my addictive tendencies was cake! Unbeknownst to me I had opened the floodgates to my addiction.

The next day we headed out to travel to our next destination. We decided to stop at a restaurant we had never tried for lunch. I was doing great. My food was healthier choices. I was enjoying myself and staying on plan.   I actually had no intention of ordering dessert!   That was, I had no intention until I saw the wait staff walk by shaking a brown paper bag. The aroma that was wafting from the paper bag was divine! I craned my neck to follow them as they carried the bag to a table of diners. I was intrigued! The first chance I got I asked my waiter exactly what was in the bag. "Donuts," was the reply. "Freshly fried donuts dropped into a bag with cinnamon sugar." The shaking motion was the waiter distributing and coating the donut with the sugary goodness. I was hooked. It had been so long since I had a donut. I had already caved the night before, why not have just a wee indulgence today also. It's was still kind of a wedding treat, right?

I was right. The donuts were incredible. The dessert at dinner that night was also delicious. Every meal that came up I couldn't resist the dessert menu. It was like the floodgates had opened up with that single piece of cake and I was powerless against the onslaught!

This is in no way anything against that bride. The choice was mine. And she was right. ONE piece of cake at a wedding was not going to ruin my efforts to maintain / lose weight.   The problem was very much mine in that I lost control of myself and couldn't stop at just one dessert. That 10-day vacation was full of tasty desserts!   I started strong with my exercise! But the desire to exercise decreased while my craving for sweet treats increased!

When vacation was over and I got back home I stepped onto the scale. I had gained 10 pounds. The one piece of lucky wedding cake was my downfall!

Miscellaneous

Legs of Steel

The weekend trip to Manassas, VA was a cold weekend. We knew that we would be spending as much time inside as possible. The first night we stayed at our hotel, ordered pizza and watched some movies on the television. It was a relaxed time, with lots of time to talk and laugh together.

As we lay on the bed together, Jason caressed my legs and started to talk about the muscles evident in them. My legs were wrapped around him and I gave him a light squeeze. Jason's eyes lit up and immediately he said, "That felt good, squeeze me as tight as you can." Giggling a bit, I complied. I tightened my legs around his chest and I squeezed.

"POP"

Ok, in fairness, I didn't hear or feel the pop. But he did. ON NO!!!! I immediately felt horrible!!! I had hurt my boyfriend. Yes, it was in jest but I had physically hurt him.

His pain was more than he let on I believe. It hurt to press upon his chest. It hurt for him to take a deep breath. It still hurt when we hiked a few days later and his footsteps would hit the ground with any kind of force. Yeah. I felt guilty and upset!!!!!! I didn't mean to hurt him!

Even upset, I did get a giggle. because really, who can say that they accidentally broke their boyfriends' ribs through an innocent request of his?

It did heal and I vowed to never heed his request to squeeze as hard as I could!

A good weigh in

It was a normal morning. I woke up and immediately headed to the bathroom. I quickly conducted my business and stripped down to hop into the shower. Every day before I stepped into the shower I hopped on the scales. I was still half-asleep when I stepped on the scales that day. I lazily looked down at the numbers on the scales and immediately I was wide-awake! I could not believe the number on the scale! There had to have been a mistake! I stepped off and then stepped back on. The number was exactly the same! For the first time in my adult life, I saw a one as my first number! I was in onderland! I let out an excited scream and threw on my clothes! I had to share this news! I rushed toward the door. I got to the door and turned the handle to open the door. The knob turned. In my rush, I started to run through the door by pushing as soon as I felt the knob turn.

Well let me tell you, the doorknob had turned but the door had not fully unlatched! My face flew up against the door. My glasses were literally knocked off my face. I was smashed up against that door flatter than a pancake. What a spectacle I must have made. It actually hurt!

I did not let that stop me though. I finally got the door open. As I opened it, I saw my husband (ex) coming flying toward me. I had made such a loud racket when I had crashed into the door that he had had come to investigate the cause of the noise.

I did not know what to say at first. Should I tell him what the noise had been. Should I tell him that I had run face first into the door. Or should I proudly announce the reason I had run headlong into a closed door and that was I had made it to onederland!

I opted for the biggest and most important piece of information and that was my weight! I could not wait a second longer to share the good news of my weigh in!

The Pink Ladies

I had an amazing group of coworkers! We got down to business and got our work done. But when we had any downtime, we laughed and had so much fun. These women were awesome. I was happy in my group and I was happy with myself. Even though I weighed over 300 pounds, I did not see myself as overweight. I was just a gal in her early 30's enjoying life and having fun with her coworkers. Our small group was dubbed "The Pink Ladies". It started simply because a manager had jokingly called us the pink ladies, but we played it up. We got a small Pink Christmas tree that we kept up at our desks. We had pink everything. I think we even at one point had a pink wig that we wore on occasion for a laugh. It was a fun group of women!

 In retrospect, it should come as no surprise that one day the conversation turned to weight loss. I sat and listened to the conversation but I did not participate. I honestly had nothing to give to the conversation. I had never dieted! I had never tried to lose weight. In fact, I   did not see myself as having any kind of weight problem, even though at the time I was morbidly obese.   There had been about two times in my life when I had dropped a few pounds. However, they had happened accidentally. One time I lost weight due to some extraordinary stress and the other time was due to ramping up my activity level. (Most people gain weight in college. Not me, I lost weight due to being so active!) Since I didn't have any problem with my weight, I just sat quietly and listened to the conversation swirl around me.

Before I knew it, this group of women had decided that we were going to have a weight loss challenge.   I sat there planning to cheer everyone along on their quest to lose weight. I had no plans to join the group. However, every one of those other pink ladies automatically assumed that I would be part of their weight loss challenge. They saw the truth that I could not see. I was seriously overweight and needed this weight loss challenge more than anyone. Before I knew it, I was part of a weight loss challenge! Me! The gal who had never even uttered the word diet! No way! No How!   But yet, there I was.

I would love to say that the weight loss challenge that the Pink Ladies had was a rousing success. However, it died a rather quick death. It was so quick that we had our initial weigh in but never had another one.   It fizzled out with no weight loss.

There was one benefit of this short-lived challenge.   That challenge is what spurred me onward to lose weight. It encouraged me to actually look at myself and recognize that I needed to get my health in line. That was the start of my weight loss journey.

Abe's Babe

I was consistently running on the Antietam Battlefield National Park. On Sunday mornings I would go and run a few miles super early. I timed it so that I could finish my run in time to meet with a friend to go for a walk.   It was a perfect opportunity to get a run in and our walks were a great cool down (and gab session). However, one Sunday morning I got more than I bargained for. I met a celebrity.

Ok, maybe he wasn't exactly a celebrity!

I was running and doing my thing one Sunday morning in the middle of summer. I was happy to be out early to beat the heat for my run. But let me tell you, it was already hot! It was so hot that I seriously thought that I was delusional at one point! Ok, maybe that was because I saw a historical celebrity right before me on the battlefield!

I am not kidding you. Right here before my eyes, in the middle of Bloody Lane (A historical site within the Antietam National Battlefield) stood Abe Lincoln!   Was it a ghost, because after all; The Bloody Lane is supposed to be one of the most haunted places on the battlefield. Or was I just delusional?

It turns out that it was not a ghost. Nor was I delusional. There were a group of men touring the battlefield that early Sunday morning. (Which is odd in itself, because you don't usually get tourists at 6AM on the Battlefield.)   Most of the men were dressed like normal tourists. However, one rather tall gentleman was dressed as Abraham Lincoln. Yes, he was just touring the battlefield dressed as a dead president!

Even as I write this, years later I have to sit back and question my sanity. Did that really happen or did I dream it up?   But I know that it happened. You see, I couldn't believe my eyes and asked if I could have my picture taken with Abe. "Abe" was all too happy to comply, even with my stinky sweaty post run body.   That way day that I became one of "Abe's Babes" as his friends all laughed while they were taking the picture and called me "Abe's Babe".

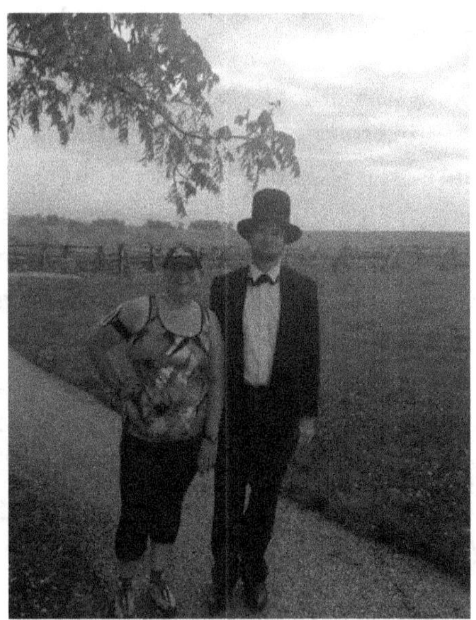

Bewildering Pain

I was having amazing success with my weight loss. I was consistently losing and I was totally focused on what I was eating and I was keeping things in check. Things were going amazingly well and I was navigating all food situations like a champ. One day I went to the local restaurant, Waffle House. I sat down determined to keep it under control and started to scan the menu. My heart sank and I was filled with defeat. I knew what the points/calories would be for the meal that I wanted and it would take up about half of my daily allowance, just for breakfast! What was I going to do? Something drew my eye down to the area for waffles. I pulled out my calculator and realized that I could have a waffle with sugar free syrup for just a fraction of points/calories. SOLD!   I ordered that waffle and I was extremely proud of myself.   I ate my breakfast and headed to work. I had only grabbed an apple for a midafternoon snack since I had gone to Waffle House for my big hearty breakfast. Except, I hadn't eaten a big hearty breakfast! It was about 2 in the afternoon when I started to feel sick. I felt so weird! My stomach was hurting so bad! I was worried to eat or drink anything because I felt so badly, but I was thirsty so I took a wee sip of water. I felt a bit better, but the pain came back very quickly. I remained worried and a bit later took another wee sip of water to assuage my thirst. Once again, my stomach felt better…for about 5-10 minutes.   I should probably be embarrassed to admit that it took me quite a while until I realized what was happening. I must have repeated the cycle of feel bad, sip water, feel over and over! Eventually I recognized the pattern and started to ponder this odd recurring occurrence. All of a sudden, the light bulb clicked!   I was actually hungry! My body was demanding food! I immediately ate my apple and it took care of the problem!

Ok, this may not seem like a huge amazing revelation. But for me, that was profound! For years and years, I just ate for the sake of eating; never really thinking about the fact that my body actually needs this food for nourishment in order to sustain my life. I had been simply shoveling food into my body with a wild abandon. I very rarely got to the point that my body was demanding food!   This was huge for me. It showed me that I really do need to listen to my body! It will talk to me!

Blind As a Bat

I had been weighing myself daily and I was frustrated. The scales were not moving in the right direction. For weeks they had been staying at or near the same weight, 263-264 pounds. They were not budging at all. The frustration was high. I wanted the number on the scale to change so badly. I was willing to do almost anything to have it move. I decided to not weigh myself for a few days. I needed the break from the daily disappointment. I finally stepped on the scale and low and behold it worked. Kinda! The numbers on the scales had definitely moved. But they had moved in the wrong direction! The last digit was not an 8! I had gained weight! I was so disillusioned, disappointed and disgusted!   What in the world? I got in the shower, near tears. I vowed to not let the numbers on the scale detract me from my mission to lose weight. The next day I was back on the scales with the same 8 at the end of the number. I was disappointed but at least I hadn't gained. It went on for a day or two. And then something changed.

I wear glasses. I also weigh myself right before I step into the shower. Now I don't' know about you, but I take off my glasses to shower. When I had been weighing myself, I was doing so without the benefit of my glasses. This means that I was partially blind. I was focusing so hard on the numbers. I put all my energy into seeing that final digit that would tell me what my weight was. You see, I knew the first two numbers a 26….it was the final digit that was in question. But one day, for some reason; I hopped on the scale with my glasses firmly affixed on my head. I looked at the number on the scale. I saw the 8 for sure. But with my glasses on, I was able to quickly see the whole number with no effort.   I was shocked.   I was in awe. I immediately started to laugh.

You see, I had been 163-164 pounds and when I saw the 8 at the end, I had assumed that I had popped up on the scales to 168. In fact, I had not gained weight all. I had indeed lost weight. I was actually down to 158 pounds.   I went through a week of disappointment and frustration simply because I didn't wear my glasses.

Non-Scale Victories

The Vixen

One evening I was cleaning up files on my computer and dumping pictures from some digital cameras. I like to take pictures and typically take quite a few, so this process is necessary from time to time. It was an easy task and one that I actually enjoy completing because it allows me the opportunity to go back and revisit memories through the pictures that I have taken previously. Occasionally, I would find a group of pictures in my photo files that were taken by my then husband. No problem, I would just put them in his file and move on. This night was no different. I laughed at one picture or another. I labelled, sorted and filed. All was going well. Until I saw "Her".

What was the first thing I thought when I came across the picture of "her"? My first thought was, who in the world is this? I had no clue who the woman in the picture was. As quickly as I questioned the identity of this woman, I began to assimilate that this picture had been taken by my (ex) husband because I certainly did not take a picture of a strange woman. I also quickly ascertained that the picture was taken in our business and this woman was posing in front of our equipment. Yes, Posing! How brazen! Then it hit me. My husband (at that time) had actually had a woman on our property and he actually felt it important enough to take a picture of her. On my camera!   In addition, he left the evidence on my camera!   How stupid was he! The steam began to roll from my pores. I was getting madder with each passing minute.

Through clenched teeth, I called him over to my computer. My words were clipped and short with anger, as I demanded, "Who is this woman?"   I pointed at the posing vixen on the computer screen and turned to face him as I awaited the answer to my question.

He started to laugh.

I do not rightly know what kept me from hitting him at that moment. Ok, I am not a violent person, so that is the reason. However, let me tell you, I was that angry! I think he could see the blood boiling very near the surface because he started to talk.

"MaryFran, look at the clothes. Those are your clothes!"

"Great, so she is wearing my clothes now also," I spewed with the venom that can only be found in a woman scorned. It was during my scathing response that I looked at the picture once again. My eyes widened and I moved my face closer to the screen. No, it couldn't be! Could it?

Oh yes, it could!   The posing vixen was none other than myself! I had lost so much weight that I did not recognize myself!

As a side note: Of course I look in the mirror each day, and should be able to see the changes within my body in the reflection. However, I have often talked about the fact that even at my lowest weight that I can look in the mirror and I still see the overweight MaryFran. My mind has become somewhat distorted and seeing the positive changes within myself has historically been difficult. The only time I have been able to SEE the changes is not when I look in the mirror, but rather when I see pictures of myself.

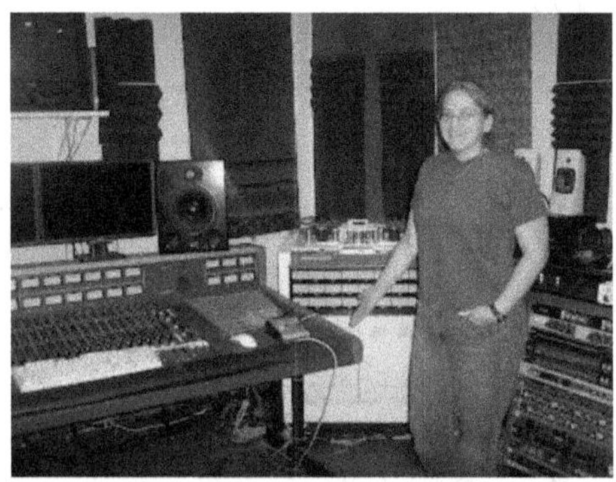

The vixen

MEOW

The sun was bright and felt warm on my skin as I walked back to the deli from the dumpster after having deposited our latest bag of garbage. I usually volunteered for trash duty because it gave me a few minutes to get outdoors during my work day. I had recently lost a lot of weight and I had a new pep in my step. I was feeling on top of the world as I strolled down the sidewalk minding my own business in this small town.

Yes, I heard the whistle. I mean seriously. How could one miss the loud catcall whistle that some men make? I did not think anything of it though and ignored it. Men do not whistle and catcall at overweight women. At least not this overweight woman. Therefore, I kept strolling lost in my own world.

"Hey you there walking on the sidewalk," I heard a voice call out. I looked around and confirmed I was the only person in sight.   I looked over at the voice to see a truck with a guy hanging out of the window. As soon as I made eye contact, he let out another catcall whistle and waved.

No, this could not be for me! However, it was and I was shocked! Yes, shock. You see I had lost a lot of weight but while I saw the numbers dropping on the scale and knew that I was wearing smaller clothes, I did not identify myself as a thin person. In my mind, I was still the grossly overweight woman who in her 35 years had never had a man whistle at her.

Only a second of time passed between the wave and my next movement. However, my mind was whirling with the surprise of having a man catcall me. I was struggling to wrap my mind around what had happened just seconds earlier and therefore I was not paying attention to where I was going and missed the half step up on the sidewalk. I stumbled and down I went.

Yes, my first catcall whistle and I fell flat on my face in shock! Literally! The truck drove on, probably laughing hysterically. I picked myself up and went back to work unscathed with no injuries. However, I had a huge smile on my face. I was not at all upset about the catcall; I was actually proud of it.

Introduction

I was blessed with awesome parents in life. Therefore, when they asked if I wanted to join them and go out to dinner I was more than happy to accept.   Our choice of restaurants was simple, as my parents loved a local diner style restaurant in a neighboring town. It did not take us long to be seated at our table and since this was a place that my parents and family frequented; we were able to place our order rather quickly. I was able to order my food wisely with my healthy lifestyle in mind. After all, I had lost a lot of weight and I wanted to keep that weight off.

We were sitting at our table waiting for our food to be prepared and brought to our table when we noticed the host seating a table of diners at the table next to us.   To our surprise, my aunt sat down at the table next to us. My parents turned to greet my aunt. We all said hello to each other and then I sat back quietly while they caught up and talked. Occasionally I would nod in agreement as part of the conversation, but as I was not close to my aunt. I did not feel any need to join in the conversation more than my occasional nod and that initial hello.

After a few minutes of conversation, my aunt looked at my father and said, "Aren't you going to introduce me to your dining companion?"   She said this as she gestured at me.

Now granted, I had not seen my aunt in a while. I had also lost a significant amount of weight in the interim. However, my own aunt did not recognize me! The look of shock on her face when my father was able to say, "This is MaryFran" was actually hysterical.

That simple phrase was a reminder of how much weight I had lost and what an amazing transformation I had enacted upon my body. In addition, let me tell you, I cannot tell you how proud I felt that night.   I was on cloud nine!

Hey it's me

It was a normal errand day for my (ex) husband and I. We had a lot of places to visit and things to do. One of our chores was a stop at our local Walmart. As we entered the store, we decided to split apart and go our own separate ways. With a quick, "I'll meet you here in about a half hour," we headed off by ourselves.

I was the first person to make it back to the reconnect destination. I was not worried or bothered, as we had set a loose timeframe. It wasn't long before I saw him amble by my cart. He totally ignored me and I could see that he was looking for something. I figured that he was still doing his shopping and stood there patiently. However, a few moments later I saw him stroll by in the other direction, still obviously looking for something. Three times he strolled by and that is when I knew that he was looking for me. "Hey Todd," I called out to bring his attention to myself. I saw him turn to look my way. We made eye contact and he turned away and continued to look for me. I had to call him two more times before his eyes and his brain connected with the knowledge that the woman calling out his name was indeed, the very same person that he was looking for.

I had lost so much weight that I was virtually unrecognizable. While he had been seeing the changes in me daily, when we were apart and his mind was elsewhere, his brain reverted to looking for and expecting to see the find the fat MaryFran. My own husband didn't recognize me due to the substantial weight loss transformation that I had undergone.

Is your Daughter Sick

For quite a few years, I would host a fourth of July party. I lived quite near the Antietam Battlefield at the time and it was the perfect place to host a party as my guests. My guests had the option to stay at my house and watch the fireworks from a distance or they could walk over to the actual battlefield and listen to the Maryland Symphony perform and watch the fireworks from a closer vantage point.

It was a fun time and each year we would always ask the same people to return with a new addition here and there. My guest list usually included my friends and family. I also included a couple of people that were close friends of my parents. On the repeat guest list was my parent's friends Dick and Eloise. I usually only saw them once a year at the party, so it was always fun for me to see them and catch up.

On the year following my most substantial weight loss period, we hosted our party as normal. I ate wisely but still thoroughly enjoyed the food, company and event. I was practicing the belief of living a healthy lifestyle in a sustainable way. I was eating everything that I wanted, just in moderation. That meant that I did have a piece of cake and I did enjoy a few higher caloric food items. Due to the way I was eating, it was not obvious to anyone that I was actually restricting my food intake at all. I just seemed like the normal 'Fat MaryFran' who was enjoying food.

It was not until the next day when my mom called me that I realized that what had been going on in the thoughts of my mom's friend the whole party.   Mom called to tell me about the phone call that she had received the next morning after the party.   Mom's friend had called to talk about me! ME! Eloise, the friend was extremely worried and wanted to ask my mom if I was sick due to my extreme weight loss.   Eloise relayed to mom about how she had watched what I was eating but did not discern anything amiss with my eating, as I seemed to be eating normally. Her only conclusion was that I had been sick and that illness had caused my substantial weight loss. My mother of course set her straight and told her that I had lost the weight the good old-fashioned way; by restricting food and ramping up the exercise.

I am so glad that my mom decided to tell me this story. I worked hard for that weight loss and to know that it was so drastic that people thought I had been sick made me feel so proud. It was an amazing feeling and reminded me of my huge accomplishment.

Who is on our Porch

I was meeting up with my parents at their house. I wasn't worried when they were not at the house when I arrived. They were out running errands but had made sure that I knew that they would be there very soon if I beat them there.   I let myself in, gave their cat a few pets, and then headed out on the porch so that I could enjoy the warm spring air while I waited for them. It wasn't long before I saw their car pull up. I waved my greeting and watched as they parked. I could see my parents in the car laughing. The laughing continued even as they got out of the car.   It turns out that I was the reason for the laughter.

As they had pulled up to the house they had seen me on their porch and my dad said, "Who is that sitting on our porch?" Apparently, before my mom could respond, I had given my wave so my dad continued "She obviously knows us since she just waved."

My mom had to remind my father that I had lost a LOT of weight and that the gal sitting on their front porch was indeed his very own daughter. My weight loss transformation was so intense that my own father had some difficulty recognizing me at the beginning.

Hershey Bar

I was working at a local deli in the town that I lived in. I had some amazing coworkers and we would have a blast during our down times.   Many days it would be three of us working for a shift during the busy summer months. One day during one of our down times, my coworker Deb decided to run next door to the town library. Russ, the other employee and myself assured her that we had everything under control. "Take your time." we called out as she walked out the door.

It was not long before Deb came back from the library with her newly checked out book. She also returned with a few 100 Calorie Hershey bars. "The librarian had a bowl of candy and told me to take one of each of you," she stated as she handed us each our small candy bar.

I looked at that candy bar as gold! It was my weigh in day at weight watchers and I did not want to eat anything unnecessary before my weigh in. No way was I going to mess that up! However, I really wanted that candy bar. I could almost taste it! I quickly decided that I would save it for after my weigh in. I was usually really hungry after the evening weigh in since the evening meeting pushed my dinner back to about 8 or 9 PM. I had it all planned out in my mind.

My coworker Russ dug right into his candy bar. It did not take long before he reached over to eat my candy bar. His words stunned me. "You don't need it, your skinny".   What? Me skinny? I started to laugh. There was no way that I was skinny.

In fact, according to the BMI index, at that point I was still at a weight where I was considered obese. I was about 10 pounds away from being categorized as simply 'overweight'.   Seriously, did my coworker still called me skinny?

Still laughing I commented and said "I'm not skinny...yet" and his remark was, "well to me you are".

His sweet-talking did not cause me to give up my candy bar. However, it did make me start to think about how I was still not seeing the amazing progress that I had made in my weight loss efforts. I had lost quite a few pounds but was not focusing on what I had lost but only what I still had to lose. I was skinny. Skinnier at least!

Look at you

I woke up early and decided to go for a walk on the Antietam Battlefield which was very near where I lived at the time. It is a gorgeous place to walk. I especially liked to walk in the early morning when the national park is not inundated with tourists, when the dew was still clinging to the crops in the field and the sun was just starting to peek out. This day was no different. It was nice to be out and about. I decided to swing through a field and cut through the visitor center parking lot to get to a different area of the battlefield. I swung around the corner and ran smack into a person that used to frequent the deli where I had previously worked. I hadn't seen this person in about a year, so it was good to see them. But the best part about seeing them for me, was their first words.

"Look at you, Skinny". I had been starting to lose my weight when I was at the deli, but I had lost a lot more weight in the following year. It must have been quite obvious! It made me feel great!   Sure, my family compliments me and I totally appreciate it. However, it really means something coming from someone that you barely know.

Skinny? Me!   I loved it!

The Thin Aunt

I was in the best shape of my life. I was running 15-20 miles a week. I was religiously going to Zumba classes. Bare minimum I went to three classes. However, whenever my work schedule allowed; I would attend back-to-back classes to make my total Zumba classes 6 for the week. I was riding my bike a few times a week. To round out my fitness regime, I was consistently working out with exercise DVD's on the days when there was no Zumba. I may not have been at my lowest weight at that time, but I was certainly the most fit I had ever been and I loved it! For the first time in my adult life, I was able to run and move and have the energy to do all of this. For the first time I was ready to be the thin aunt.

It was a Sunday afternoon and I went to my parents to spend the day with family. My brother and his family lived across the street from my parents, so it was a full family affair. Midway through the day, my brother's family decided to go to the park. Their youngest son was just learning to ride a two wheeled bike and they wanted the open field for him to practice. The two oldest kids wanted to kick around the soccer ball. I was all in! We piled in their car and off we went.

I had the time of my life! For the first time ever, I was able to be the thin aunt that had the energy to really run and play with the kids. I was able to run with the kids while we played with the soccer ball. I was able to run alongside my nephew as he worked on riding a bike without training wheels. I was able to keep up with all three of them and not feel as if I was dying!

That afternoon in the park may not have been a memory that will stick in anyone else's mind. But that day, was the day that I realized exactly how much the weight had kept me from living life to the fullest!

The little Ones

So many of the non-scale victories I have experienced during this journey aren't a big story like the ones I have just written about. They aren't a whole litany of events and circumstances. Most of my non scale victories have been small blips in time. It is the day that I got of the shower and discovered that I could wrap the towel around myself with no gap. I was completely covered. It was the moment that I realized that I could cross my legs like a lady without my leg jutting out at some weird angle. The non scale victory was huge the day I went to a store and realized that I could actually fit into clothes from regular stores and not having to go to the plus size stores or departments. Another non scale victory was the day I went to an amusement park and realized that I didn't have to turn, squeeze and contort myself to go through the turnstiles and instead just plow straight through them. Those are the non-scale victories of life. As I lost weight, it was a whole new world. Life was different each day as I discovered and experienced new non-scale victories. It is a feeling of awe and amazement and words can not describe! Little or big, non-scale victories are the biggest and grandest reward for all the hard work!

Society

Society plays a huge role in the obesity epidemic that has gripped the world. Employers feed their employees at work functions. Celebrations with family typically occur around a table with food as the centerpiece. Food is at the forefront of our world.   This structure of everyday life contributes to a person being overweight. Yet, society continues to bombard us with pictures of the 'perfect' size in magazines and tv shows. Our world puts on a pedestal the perfect body but then works to ensure that the average person struggles to achieve that goal. These messages that our society has bombarded us with trickles down into the way we react to situations, the things we say to people and the decisions we make. That trickle down affect from societal norms can have some serious repercussions.

A heavy bike for a heavy girl

It was a Sunday morning and I was so excited or my plans for the day! I was going to go to church in the morning where I would hook up with my friend. After church, we were going to grab her bike from her house, pick up some sandwiches at a local deli and we then were going to go for a bike picnic. (A bike picnic is simply putting a picnic lunch in a backpack and biking to the picnic destination, enjoying the picnic and then biking home.) It sounded like a fabulous day and I could not wait!

The morning went off as planned and shortly after church, we were on the way to her house to pick up her bike. I had a rooftop bike rack on my car and I was most familiar with loading a bike into the rack so I offered to put her bike in the rack. I went to pick up the bike and I stopped short as I lifted. That thing was HEAVY! It was at least double the weight of my bike! I looked at the bike, thinking that she had placed her backpack or full bottles of water on the bike. However, there was nothing extraneous on the bike. This bike was just plain heavy!   What in the world?

I couldn't help it. I made a comment about how heavy her bike was in comparison to mine.   My friend laughed and came back and said, "My dad was with me when I bought the bike. He wanted to make sure I bought a sturdy bike since I am a hefty girl".

My jaw dropped. What a horrible thing to say to your daughter! I am sure he meant well, but what hurtful words.   I was about the same weight as my friend, my bike was half the weight, and it was quite sturdy.   (In fact, I still have that bike and it is comfortably ridable even now, 20 some years later. I have ridden that bike when I was over 300 pounds and when I was under 200 and every pound in between.) There was no reason that this girl needed a sturdy heavy bike. That heavy bike was only holding her back and only serving to make riding a bike more difficult and not so much fun.   To want to do something repeatedly in a continual ongoing effort, the activity needs to be enjoyable not torturous!   Furthermore, continual effort is exactly what someone needs to have in order to lose the weight in order to not be so 'hefty'.

My friend did not seem to be outwardly upset but I know that those words were stuck in her head. They were slowly undermining her confidence. Those words were a self-fulfilling prophecy as she conducted herself and her life in a way to 'live up' to the expectations of being a 'hefty girl'.   Those words had the power to do quite a bit of damage!

Egging me On

I worked in a small local bank. There were only 6 of us that worked at this branch and we had a lot of fun together. When Christmas rolled around, we decided to celebrate with a nice holiday dinner that we ordered from a local restaurant. I was actually super happy with this choice because it would allow me to control what I ate. I would not be confronted with a table full of food at a potluck dinner. We were a small group, but we liked our food and we usually had enough food to feed an army (seriously, there were times we ate the leftovers for a few days)! By ordering a nice dinner from a restaurant, I would be able to choose a healthy option. I would have some control over my portion size. When what I ordered was done, I had no more food to eat. What was on my plate would be all that I would have access to eat.   Furthermore, since I knew what I was ordering a few days before the event, I was able to plan my eating for the day to accommodate for a meal that took a bigger bite out of my food budget then normal. I was absolutely tickled! I made my choice. I ordered a marinated chicken breast. I went with an extra side of steamed vegetables to replace the potato and asked for no dinner roll. I was a girl on a mission! I was so proud of myself!

The food came and my lunch was delicious. I was so on track with my weight loss efforts that I actually immediately packaged up the extra chicken breast and half the vegetables for my lunch the next day.   I could not have done any better with my choices

and actions.   I patted myself on the back for my job well done!
I had navigated an event that would have previously been a
disaster to any weight loss effort.

Then disaster struck. I am a December birthday girl. My
coworkers decided to celebrate my birthday on the same day as
our Christmas luncheon. That in itself is not a disaster. We all
have birthdays and we all celebrate. I opened up my card and
thanked everyone.   However, when I turned around, there was
a huge sheet cake decorated for my birthday. There were only
6 people that worked in this bank and they had purchased a full
sheet cake. This was not a half sheet cake, which would have
still been too big. No, they had a full sheet cake. I groaned
inwardly and said to myself: Cake, it would have to be cake!   I
was gracious on the outside and thanked them. I ohhhed and
ahhed over the cake and helped cut everyone a piece of cake,
serving everyone but myself. I held firm. I did NOT cut a piece
for myself.   A piece of cake was not in my budget. I had
stretched my food budget as tight as I could to account for the
luncheon. Cake was NOT in the budget and I was holding firm.

My coworkers did not want to accept this.   "It's your birthday
cake," they exclaimed. "You have to eat a piece of your own
birthday cake!" The started to push harder with various
comments. "Just a small piece!" "We bought this special for
your birthday." I tried to stick to my guns. I really did.
However, after a small length of time my resolve crumbled and I
agreed to a "SMALL" piece of cake. I specifically asked for a
very small sliver of cake. In my mind, I was calculating how
much it would cost me in terms of my food budget and what I
could do the rest of the day to account for this indulgence.

They were all babbling excitedly as they handed me my plate of
cake. I don't know what part of the phrase small sliver that
they didn't understand. They certainly must have used a
different unit of measurement because the slice of cake that

they set before me was easily over 5 inches square. They gave me the very best piece, if you love icing. This piece was piled high with icing roses and shells and all sorts of decorations fashioned out of icing.   It was the exact piece of cake that I would have loved, had I not been counting my food intake.

I drew in my breath. I could do this. One or two bites and then I would put the cake aside until the celebration was over. At that time, I could politely throw this mammoth piece of cake away. I took one bite. Oh, my word, did it ever taste good. The room erupted into cheers as I took my bite. I took my second bite and they started clapping. I sat the cake aside and they started hounding me to have more. The chanted various phrases. Eat more! Just another bite. Peer pressure got to me and I ate another bite. And then I ate another bite. Each time I took a bite, they cheered and clapped. It was as if I was an Olympian in a cake eating contest!   My coworker's eyes twinkled in delight as I ate. One coworker actually said "Look, I've never seen her eat anything bad...but she is doing it!"   The cheers continued until I ate the whole piece of cake.

I felt horrible. Sure, the cake tasted incredibly good but I was not used to eating that much sugar and my stomach felt it. Even worse, I felt like an emotional wreck. I had a plan. I was strong in that plan. And then in a moment of weakness, one that was filled with cheers and taunts from coworkers I caved. I had ruined my day. There was almost virtually no way that I could recover from this cake in terms of my daily caloric budget. The luncheon alone had put me to the edge of my limits. The cake had not just pushed me over the edge, it had flung me viciously over the cliff.

I sat quietly the rest of the day. In my mind, I was trying to come up with a plan of what I could eat for dinner that was, well filling but virtually point free /calorie free (this was in an era before the plethora of free foods on Weight Watchers).   I changed as much as I could, but I was still completely and utterly over budget for my food consumption for that day. I got home and tried to negate as much of that cake as I could by working out, but the damage had been done. The only thing I could do was to square my shoulders and move on without letting this slip send me into a downward spiral of unhealthy options.

The next day, I did not eat any of the leftover cake. My coworkers all had some, but I held firm. One of my coworkers privately came to me and apologized for her participation in the frenzy that had encouraged me to eat the cake. She said that she got home and thought about it and felt horrible when she realized what they had actually done. She was the only one. Everyone else continued to taunt and encourage me to eat the leftover cake during the next few days. I did not eat any of the leftover cake. My coworkers all had some, but with the encouragement of that one coworker, I held firm!

New Year Extravaganza

We were heading into New Year's Eve and Jason and I were planning on a little get away. We were so excited to ring the New Year in as a couple. The place that we were staying at had a kitchen and we were planning on eating in and enjoying the amenities and our time together. We had no desire to be out in the craziness of a New Year's Eve! Our food was packed and we were ready to go, with one minor exception. Dessert. It was New Year's Eve! Of course, we needed dessert!

As we talked and prepared to head to our destination, we discussed possible options for a dessert. We rattled off different options. Cinnamon Rolls or cookies? Cake or Ice cream? How about donuts! Once we said donuts, we were hooked. Donuts it would be. We decided to go to locally owned grocery store near where we lived to pick up our sweet treat, as we were enamored with their donuts. We were both quite satisfied with our decision and as soon as we were done packing the car, we headed out the door on our way to the grocery store and onward to our fun getaway.

The grocery store was not crowded and we were feeling confident as we walked toward the bakery. The grocery store actually frequently sold out of donuts. We had not come up with a backup plan so the low crowd was a good sign! We rounded the corner and the holy mecca of donuts was before us! I swear, the angels sang the song hallelujah in my ear as the aroma of hundreds of donuts wafted over my nose. They had a lot of donuts left. Even better, they had the donuts that we wanted! Luck was with us! We are creatures of habit, so it did not take us long fill up our box of donuts. Just a half dozen, for the two of us. We were not done shopping yet. So, we kept walking through the bakery area. That is when we saw it. An Apple Harvest cake. Jason's jaw dropped and he started to talk about how he used to get those cakes years earlier. He rhapsodized about the filling that was sandwiched between three moist layers of cake. I swear that I could actually see him drool when he mentioned the thick layer of caramel icing that covered the top of the cake. I could see that he wanted the cake and he wanted it bad. I encouraged him, "Go ahead and get it!" He was hesitant, due to the 6 donuts we held in our hands. But seriously, it was New Years Eve! I reminded him that it was a holiday! With that reasoning, it was a no brainer. We got that cake!   Then I saw my downfall. Brownies with Peanut butter Icing. My mouth watered! Ohhh my word, it looked good. I could almost taste it! I also hesitated, but Jason turned my words right back around. It was a special holiday after all! Yes, we got the brownies also. Luckily, we stopped at that and didn't add any more desserts to our cart. But seriously, that was enough!

We drove to our hotel and Jason continued to talk about this apple harvest cake. I could not wait to try it but I showed restraint. We had already eaten dinner and settled into our room for a quiet night together before we cracked open the desserts. I headed for my brownies first. The taste was divine! I savored each bite! However, what about those donuts? I had purchased donuts in my favorite donut flavors and I had been so looking forward to them. I ate my first pick donut. It was amazing. I ate my next donut. Ohhh, it was good. And I stopped. Yes, I ate two donuts and a lot of brownies BEFORE I stopped. But I did eventually stop!

The night was still young. We sat around and watched movies and talked and enjoyed each other's company. It was a fabulous New Year's Eve! I was loving every minute of it. As we got closer to midnight, I was ready to celebrate a little bit. I don't drink alcohol often, but I had brought the makings for some amaretto sours, my favorite drink to order. I made myself a drink and looked longingly at my final donut. I couldn't withstand the draw of the donut! It was New Years Eve and I decided to live on the edge. I decided to eat that last donut. I finished it before the ball dropped and I was rather full from my plethora of sweet treats.

But what about that Apple harvest cake? I had totally forgotten about the cake! "You have to at least try a wee little piece," Jason said when we realized that I hadn't even tried the cake. I figured that I could squeeze in some more dessert. Always room for dessert, right?   I cut myself a wee tiny piece of cake. It was bliss! Jason was right! The cake was delicious! Heavenly white creamy filling sandwiched between layers of moist apple cake and smothered with a caramel icing. It was super rich but also super tasty. My little sliver was definitely not enough. I went back for more! This time I cut a generous portion of cake. With each bite of the cake, I could feel myself getting fuller. Sickeningly full. However, I finished that cake right as the ball dropped!

We kissed and it was not long before we were headed to bed. My night of gluttony was over. Or was it?

I woke up the next morning and immediately knew something was wrong. My stomach was in an uproar! I moaned and headed to the bathroom, confident that a visit to the porcelain throne would ease the discomfort in my body. But no, it made no difference! I went back to bed and curled up in a ball. I was in misery. I swear sweat beads were forming on my head as I struggled with the overwhelming urge to upchuck every bite of my previous night's food fest.   It was horrible.   Jason began to move around and get ready to face the day. Not me. I laid in that hotel bed in absolute misery! I tried to take a hot shower to ease the pain in my body. But that didn't work and I found myself back in bed shortly after I got out of the shower. I can't even put to words how awful I felt.

We put all of our plans for the day on hold and I laid in bed until the last possible minute before our check out time. As time went by, I could feel myself slowly feeling not quite as queasy but I was still feeling the effects when we left the hotel. It was a holiday and our plans had been scrubbed so we drove the most scenic route home. We were in my car and typically I would drive, but not that day. I was too focused on not tossing my cookies. Slowly throughout the afternoon, I began to feel better. We arrived back to our town about 5 or 6 in the evening and we started to discuss dinner, but I was still STUFFED from all of those desserts and chose to not eat!

I can honestly say that the New Year Eve extravaganza of food was the sickest I have ever made myself from eating too much. Sure, I've overeaten and felt the effects for an hour or two. Sure, I've eaten before and not been hungry for 6, 8 or 10 hours. But never before have I been that ill from eating too much!

Fast Food Eating

I was in the drive through of a fast-food restaurant and ready to order. I had looked at my food budget and had planned my meal carefully. I was determined to stay within my food budget. The worker was very nice as they took my order. I ordered a sandwich and a drink. Nothing more nothing less. The worker was honestly just trying to help me when she advised that I could get the meal deal and save money while also getting French fries. I am sure there are plenty of people that try to order less food because they do not have the money to buy a full meal. That was not the case with me that day. I did not want the French fries. I did not have the room in my food budget to eat them that day. For me, it had nothing to do with money. I told the worker no and she was flabbergasted. She kept arguing that I was spending more money by not ordering the French fries. I knew that and I am a penny pincher so it was quite difficult for me to say no. That is exactly what I did; I told her that I was ok paying more but that I did not really want the French fries. She did not want to accept no as an answer, she kept at it...hammering the point across. Eventually

I asked if I could order the meal but they not put the fries in the bag. That sounded like a valid solution, right? However, of course that was not a valid solution; not to the fast-food joint. They were unable to do that. I knew that if those fries were in my bag that I would eat them. Finally, I had to get almost mean and firm and say, "I will pay whatever you charge me but I only want a sandwich in my bag and a drink in my hand". I felt horrible for being so firm and mean, but I was not going to let French fries derail me, not that day at least. Once again, society has made it a better financial decision to eat poorly.

Programmed to Feed

The email came from my friend. I was honestly a bit jealous! Her employer was doing a challenge. It was a 10,000-step challenge. It was going to be an awesome program that would last a few months. It would include motivational events and prizes. The event kicked off with a breakfast and inspirational speaker. How awesome! Except that the breakfast was donuts. Not exactly a healthy breakfast. We laughed about how it was a program aimed at being healthy but they weren't feeding them healthy foods. She used her willpower and avoided the landmine of the unhealthy breakfast that day. But it made me think about our society.

Our society is programmed to feed. Do you want to boost moral? Feed everyone. Do you want to make a meeting more upbeat? Provide food. I have been to countless meetings and events for work. If the meeting is close to breakfast there will most undoubtedly be a box of donuts sitting on the table. Afternoon meeting? Why yes that tray of cookies looks amazing! Sandwich trays, ice cream, bagels, candy; you name it… they offer.   It's not just meetings. I've worked with companies that reward with food. If the employees are doing good, they cater in lunch. I've even been given candy as a thank you. It is programmed into our society. Food is the key to happiness…. or so they think!

But does that food really bring you long term happiness? I would much prefer an extra 15-minute break! Maybe give us an extra day off. Even a gift card for $5 would work!

Wardrobe Malfunctions

I can't even begin to remember all of the wardrobe malfunctions I have encountered along this journey. My size was ever changing. My clothes were frequently too big. I was learning how to navigate different body shapes and different activities. There was bound to be issues with my clothes and boy oh boy where there ever!

Wedding Woes

I was excited! I was going to go to a wedding of a gal that I had babysat many years earlier. She had been teaching in a mission school in the Philippines and had met her husband there. It had been ages since I had seen her and she had not seen me since I started to lose weight.   I was feeling confident and excited to go to this wedding.   To really get the true gist of what happened, I need to back track in time to about a month or two prior to the wedding.

A few months prior to the wedding, I decided to go through my clothes closets and clear out everything that was super big on me. I had been losing weight steadily and many of my clothes in the closet were too big. I tried on every item of clothing. I had quite a collection of clothes that were too big when I was done. My closet wasn't totally empty. I had four pairs of dress pants left when I was done with my purge mission. I had two that fit perfectly and two pairs that were just a wee bit tight. I knew that I had this wedding to attend in the coming months so I closed the closet door on those four pairs of pants satisfied that I would have something to wear to the event.   I removed all of those fat clothes from the house. I was done with them!

Luckily for me, I was working a job where I just needed jeans and tee-shirts! It was fabulous! It also meant that I did not look in the closet until the morning of the wedding.

The morning of the wedding rolled around and I was busy with stuff around the house. I had thought about the clothes that were left in my closet and knew what I was going to wear, so I was not too concerned about getting ready. It was about an hour or so before I had to leave the house that I headed to the closet to grab the pants that I had decided to wear. I slipped on the clothes. When I say slipped, I mean dove in. They were huge! I looked like I was a clown in baggy billowing pants.   I tried the next pair. It was just as bad. My bottom half looked like a big round ball because the hem of the pants rested on the floor and the pants just ballooned out. I tried the next pair with the same results. Panicked I tried the last pair and stood there in utter disbelief.

On one hand, I was super excited! I had just shrunk out of ALL of my dress pants!
What an amazing non-scale victory! Go me!   On the other hand, I was in a state of panic. The clock was ticking! I had a little less than an hour before I needed to leave the house to go to this wedding. I had nothing to wear to a wedding. The only clothes that fit me in the house were blue jeans! Holy cow what was I going to do! Suddenly I had a crazy thought. What about that old box of clothes up in the attic?   It was a box of old clothes from high school and college. Clothes that I absolutely loved and could not bear to get rid of due to the memories that they held. The idea that there would be something in that bin was insanely crazy, preposterous really; but I had no choice. The clock was ticking. I had to find something other clothes that looked like a clown outfit to wear to this wedding. I headed up to the attic.

Let me tell you, I tore through that box of clothes. Much of it
was worthless for my current cause. Miraculously there was
one thing in that box that worked and it was not blue jeans!
What I found was a jeans style cut but the fabric was a soft-
brushed denim the color of a deep wine. I was able to pair that
up with a solid tee shirt that fit and a dress shirt (loose) over
that. It was not exactly wedding attire, but it was my only
option. Whew...crisis averted!

The pockets

Shrinking out of your clothes is a costly venture. Every twenty
to thirty pounds of weight loss would cause me to need to get
all new clothes. It was an exciting problem to have, but also a
costly problem. The biggest issue was with pants. Shirts can be
loose and while they may not look as nice big and baggy, it is
not a problem.   Pants on the other hand, wearing them big and
baggy can be a problem.   I got into a routine. I would buy two
or three pairs of pants in my current size. That would give me
only a half week or clothes. Sometimes I would just wash and
wear the same thing over, but most frequently I would also
have days where I would wear a pair of big and baggy pants. I
had one pair in particular that while big didn't look too horrible
on me due to the style and cut. I would wear them pretty
frequently, even though I had gotten to the point that I could
put them on and take them off without having to unbutton or
unzip them. They would slip on and off with ease. How
convenient!

I was wearing these pants one day while I was working at a bank
as a teller. I was going about my day and not thinking about my
pants. The day was going splendidly. It was mid afternoon
when I had a customer come in and ask to get into their safe
deposit box. No problem. I grabbed my keys and ushered them

into the vault. As I waited for them to sign the log book, I went to slip the keys and my hands into my pockets. Except my hands wouldn't easily slide in. I tried it again and the same thing. I tried the other side and it just wasn't happening. I was utterly confused! What in the world. My fingers would slide in to just about my first knuckle and then meet with resistance. I wiggled my fingers into the pocket a bit deeper trying to figure out what in the world was the matter. And that is when I noticed that my hands would slide in.... backwards! I looked down and my jaw dropped. I had just slipped on my pants that morning when I got dressed for work. I had been slipping them on and off all day long when I went to the bathroom. I had NEVER noticed that the zipper and button were in the back! I had been wearing my pants backwards all day long! No one ever said a word to me! I was a bit mortified and embarrassed. I wanted to fix this problem immediately but I couldn't leave the customer in the vault! I brazened it out and completed the job at hand. It wasn't until they were heading out of the bank before I could make a beeline to the bathroom to put my pants on the right way! Ooops!

Commando at the Gym

I went to get dressed. I opened up my underwear drawer and out of habit just started to grab the top pair off the pile. I stopped and started to think. You see, the last few time that I had gone to the gym, I'd had a bit of a problem. You see......well......to put it bluntly my underwear would ride in ways that they shouldn't ride. OK OK OK, I've gotten wedgies! Exercise wedgies you might say. So anyway, I was looking into the drawer contemplating what pair would best serve my purposes and NOT ride in an uncomfortable manner. And that is when I got a grand idea! I've never been much of a 'commando' girl myself...but I started to think. If I just put on my exercise pants and skipped the underwear...well...there would be nothing to ride improperly! What a grand idea!!!! I couldn't believe my stroke of genius! So off to the gym I went. I did have a momentary thought of what would happen if my pants ripped out at the seam. But I put that thought out of my mind! I entered the gym. I immediately headed to the elliptical machine. I set myself up and started my workout. I was amazed at how wonderful my 'plan' was working. I felt no uncomfortable 'riding'. It was great. I pushed myself on the elliptical and my time on that machine eventually ended. From there I moved over to an upright exercise bike. I rode HARD....sweat was dripping. I was going gang busters ahead and knocking fat off of my body! It wasn't until I hit my cool down that I looked down. Now don't ask me why I looked down and noticed the crotch of my pants. But that is exactly what I did. Ohhh my word, it looked like I peed myself. Apparently, the underwear acts as a wick and collects the sweat and keeps it from pooling in the crotch of my pants! With no underwear, the sweat had just dripped and collected in a pool right in my crotch area. I had to walk out of the gym and across the parking lot looking like I had peed my pants!!!! NEVER again will I go commando to the gym!!!

On a Whim

I was out and had a few minutes to kill before meeting my friend so I decided to walk through an overstock store (Everything is five dollars or below). I was just perusing the merchandise when I spotted a pair of pants. It was a pair of flannel pants. Nothing too fancy, but something that a person always needs in the winter. I looked at them and actually walked by them at first because I was sure that I could not fit into any clothes at a regular store. I had to go to what I termed "the fat ladies store" to buy my clothes. That thought was so ingrained in my head that I walked by those pants three of four times before I realized that I had lost a fair amount of weight and maybe, just maybe; I could fit into a pair.

I scurried back to the shelf of lounging flannel pants. I was going to try it! I was fingering them and pondering the sizes. As I lost the weight, I honestly had no clue what size I was. It really was a guessing game when I was buying clothes. I had to try on everything as every part of my body changed sizes (from ring size to shoe size and everything in between. That day, I was convinced that I should get the size XXL. Only a few months earlier even that size would have been excessively small for me. I was sure that the XXL would still be a tight fit.

However, something happened to my thinking. I do not know what overcame me. I have no clue what my thought process was. I just could not help myself. I turned away from the XXL and picked up the XL. I had absolutely no hope of fitting into that size. I was not an XL girl. I was a big girl and wearing single X Large was incomprehensible! The only thing in my head was that someday I would be able to wear them. I did not dither and want to purchase the flannel lounging pants. I did not think about them again until I got home.

I pulled the pants out of the shopping back later that day when I finally got home. I looked at them and practically snorted at the thought that I had actually deigned to buy an extra-large instead of the larger size that I most definitely needed. I was getting ready to carry them into the closet where they would sit in a box and await for my body to shrink a bit more so that I could wear them. However, before I could do that, a thought niggled in my head. "Maybe you should try them on to see how close you are to fitting into those size extra-large pants."

I opened the package and slid the soft flannel pants up my legs. My eyes got wide because the pants were sliding right up with no resistance! My mind was spinning with the thought that

maybe I was closer to wearing them then I had thought!   I kept
pulling the pants up and they went right over my stomach. The
elastic waistband on the pants popped comfortably into place.
They were actually loose! In fairness, they were not so loose
that I would have needed another size lower. But they were
loose and a bit baggy and quite comfortable to wear and lounge
around the house in!

I do not know what possessed me to buy the smaller size that
day! However, I am so glad that I did! It is such an amazing
feeling when you can fit into the next size smaller clothes!

Size Small

I was out with my mom and dad for lunch. We were enjoying
our food and company. But I was having a serious problem.
Every time I stood up, I had to hitch up my pants. They weren't
in danger of totally falling off. They were just not fitting right
and sagging, a whole bunch. (Seriously, what a fabulous
problem to have! woo hooo!) My mom was the first to
comment on my wardrobe malfunction by saying, "put on a
belt, girl". I just laughed and said...SURE, If I had one. She looked
at me in disbelief before she said, "You've got belts"   I had to
answer and explain to her that yeah, I do have belts....ones that
I wore when I was 300 plus pounds. I put them on now...and
they wrap around me practically the whole way twice! She
didn't have a comeback to that. So I just kept hiking up my
pants!

 The very next day I was with my mom at the mall. We were
waiting in line at American Eagle Outfitters to pay for a
purchase. I looked at the display beside us and low and behold
it was a rack of belts! I honestly had no intention of buying a
belt. I was planning to keep hitching my pants up until I bought
a pant size that fit me better! However; I decided to try them
on. I automatically reached for a large. The Large was way too

big. What? I am a large girl! However, the ends were flopping and hanging so far down. I couldn't believe that I needed the next size down, but I went for it.   I tried on the S-M Yeah, it fit...with room to spare. It was not even on the last hole or anything! I was laughing...I held up the belt and showed mom the size. I wasn't a solid size medium yet in my clothes purchases. I was just starting to fit into size medium. But I fit into a small/Medium belt. It was a SMALL-MEDIUM! Yeah, I bought it! In fairness, I liked it before I put it on. I also really did need a belt. But most definitely it was purchased because it was <u>SMALL</u>/medium!

The least expected

I was a losing weight machine. My clothes had gotten loose and literally fallen off. I bought new clothes, and they were also loose. I was doing amazing! Even more amazing is that I was losing all this weight while I was working in the restaurant industry! I was on top of my game and my efforts were showing!   They were showing everywhere, even where I least expected.

It was a normal day at the deli where I worked. We were rushing around preparing food and waiting on customers. I was thinking about nothing other than the job at hand.   That is until I hear a clink.   It was a delicate sound and not very loud. I'm honestly quite lucky that I not only heard it, but that it registered in my mind. But I did hear it.   And somehow my mind registered exactly what it was!   I called out to my coworkers and all movement stopped behind the deli counter where we were working.   Within seconds we were all on our hands and knees looking for the sound of the mysterious clink. Customers were peaking over the bar looking from their

vantage point in an effort to help.   Luckily, we found the source
of the clinking noise very quickly!

What was the noise?   My engagement ring and wedding band.
I had known that they were feeling a bit loose. But I had
dropped a bit more weight and the rings had gotten to the point
that if I simply held my hands straight down that the rings
would fall off my fingers

Each time I read this collection of stories I am filled with a sense
of pride mingled with a desire to laugh. Life is funny and throws
the craziest things at us. Seriously, my toaster was a coffin;
that's crazy! There will be moments that we falter. There will
be good. There will be bad. But through it all we need to learn
to embrace the crazy. We need to learn to accept that the tales
from the scales will be full of ups and downs. It isn't all rosy but
it is all part of this fabulous thing that we call life! Laugh, love
and live your life through it all and you will be successful!